The Path to Pain Control

Also by Meg Bogin:
The Women Troubadours

The Path
to Pain Control

Meg Bogin

Houghton Mifflin Company · Boston · 1982

Library of Congress Cataloging in Publication Data

Bogin, Meg.
    The path to pain control.

    Bibliography: p.
    Includes index.
    1. Pain — Prevention.   2. Pain — Chemotherapy.
I. Title.
RB127.B63   616′.0472   81–6822
ISBN 0–395–31287–6   AACR2

Printed in the United States of America

D   10 9 8 7 6 5 4 3 2 1

The author is grateful to Little, Brown and Company for permission to quote from *The Complete Poems of Emily Dickinson*, edited by Thomas H. Johnson. Copyright 1914, 1929, 1942 by Martha Dickinson Bianchi; copyright © 1957 by Mary L. Hampson.

NOTE

The information contained in Chapter 9 is based on research and recommendations of responsible medical sources. Because drug reactions are highly individual, each reader is strongly urged to check with a physician before making any change in the use of a particular medication. No one should commence taking any drug, or discontinue a prescribed drug regimen, without consulting a physician.

To Karuna Thompson

To insure oneself from hurt
is to insure oneself from growth.
GEORG GRODECK
Book of the It

Contents

Acknowledgments

Many people have helped make this book a reality. To Laura Dearborn and Bill Dasheff, who saw the first scribbled outline and gave the first all-important words of encouragement, I owe my very first words of thanks. To Carol Liebner, who next picked up the thread, secondary but no less profound acknowledgment is due. My agent, Diane Cleaver, set the wheels in motion and has been a magnificent, vigilant, diligent driver ever since.

Without the women of my Illness Support Group many of the ideas expressed in these pages would not have seen the light, because I would not have had the courage and belief to continue on the path.

Margaret Cook is the healthiest ill person I know and, at eighty-five, my most venerable teacher in matters of body and soul.

Juliene Berk has been a source of literate and literary delight; I hope she finds this book as robust as she might like.

I would also like to thank the medical experts who kindly read portions of the manuscript and offered cogent criticism: Dr. Joan Borysenko, Dr. Eric J. Cassell, Dr. Lilly Engler, and Dr. Herbert A. Schreier. To Dr. Robert Kaiko, assistant professor of pharmacology at Cornell University Medical Center and associate, Analgesic Studies Section at Memorial Sloan-Kettering Institute for Cancer Research, special thanks are due for his extraordinary patience and generosity in explaining basic pharmacology to a total novice.

Besides those already mentioned, I thank the following friends and sharp readers who fine-combed the manuscript for syntax, sensitivity, and scientific and social accuracy: Marge and Peter Albertson, Ruth and George Bogin, Eva Kollisch, Joan Nestle, Mildred Sklar, and my editor, Anita McClellan.

Finally, my very deepest thanks go to the men and women who shared with me their own intimate experience of chronic pain. I promised anonymity, so none of you is named. I can only hope that this book repays your confidence by reflecting the full dimension of your wisdom and struggle.

Introduction

Whoever you are — whether you are young, middle-aged, or old, male or female, employed or unemployed, disabled by your physical condition or relatively able — chances are that if you are reading this book it is because you are in pain, either at this very moment or a good deal of the time. Pain is enough of a presence in your life to have you looking for answers. Like me, you may have lived through months or even years of severe pain, put your trust in a series of fine doctors, tried all sorts of remedies, and become well acquainted with, if not dependent on, painkillers. Like anyone who has had to face the experience of protracted pain, you have probably felt trapped, disillusioned, inadequate, and desperate for a way out. You may have turned your desperation inward, hoping to hide your suffering from those around you and feeling increasingly cut off, or you may have begun to unload it on family and friends, creating a sea of tension around you. Whatever your story, it may help to know that you are not alone.

Millions of people throughout this country and around the world are in pain right this minute. You may feel, as I

did when I was first in pain, that other people — those un-
told millions out there — have some special knack for coping that you yourself are lacking. Nothing could be further
from the truth. Based on my own experience and on the
extensive interviews and research I did in the course of writing this book, I can assure you that saints and mystics are
few and far between. Most people find pain one of the
toughest, most wearing, most demoralizing, and most challenging experiences of their entire lives. I was no exception.

In fact, it was the very wretchedness of chronic pain and
the difficulty I had holding my life together with pain as a
pervasive presence that led me to the path of study and
exploration that evolved into this book. *The Path to Pain
Control* is the result of a long process of self-analysis, psychotherapy, research, interviewing, and hundreds of hours
of physical pain during which I had what I like to call the
leisure to try out all sorts of techniques, many of which
have become a part of my daily life and which are described
in the pages that follow. The path I set out on several years
ago in desperation enabled me to reduce my pain dramatically and to develop a long-term strategy for coping. But
this is not, strictly speaking, a personal story.

My path to pain control took me out of my own suffering,
to medical libraries and textbooks, to conferences and panels
about chronic pain, to men and women in a broad range
of health professions — nurses and neurosurgeons, acupuncturists and hypnotists, physical therapists and psychiatrists
— who deal with chronic pain in their daily practice. Most
important of all, it took me to several dozen men and women
with chronic pain who generously shared with me their observations and experience, their trials, triumphs, and tribu-
lations. I spoke to city and country dwellers, professors and
factory workers, health technicians, a beautician, psychologists, miners, secretaries, writers, a union organizer, a painter,

a social worker, and a retired teacher. Some had arthrit several had been hurt in car accidents; several had been jured on the job; three were veterans; several had chronic back problems and some had migraines; two had been hurt in sports.

All of them were strangers to me when we first began to talk; by the end of an hour we were comrades in a struggle that no one on the outside can ever fully understand. Most of the people I interviewed were doing well by the standards of the outside world; most were working, and most were keeping up a brave enough front. But what a complex inner world they shared with me! From these extraordinary conversations I learned that chronic pain transcends the categories of particular illnesses or injuries: whatever its cause, it creates in each of us a turbulent, ongoing struggle that is immediately recognizable to anyone who has lived with pain for an extended length of time. My own story is typical of those that others shared with me.

I first began to experience intense pain in the fall of 1977. I consider myself a strong, resourceful person, but in retrospect I can see how totally unprepared I was for the experience that lay in store for me. In October 1977 my legs suddenly became weak and unsteady and I began to have difficulty going up and down stairs. My gait became a lurch and my legs felt as if they had lead weights attached to them. I was twenty-seven years old and felt seventy-five. After a week my legs were aching so much I couldn't sleep — I who had never had insomnia, who had always slept like a log. I called a friend with a thirty-year history of arthritis, who told me to take aspirin around the clock. I did. Nothing happened. Ten days after the onset of the first symptoms the aches turned into full-blown, agonizing pain. I was terrified.

I went to a doctor who diagnosed rheumatism. He gave

me a low-grade painkiller that had no effect. This was the beginning (although I didn't know it then) of a string of visits to different internists and specialists in the hope that someone would take one look at me and say, "Oh, you have X disease" — something nice and benign and easy to treat — and press the magic button that would end the pain. Many doctors later, after a long search for a diagnosis and cure, I finally realized that with all that doctors can do, pressing magic buttons isn't one of them. I now know that I have a rare inflammatory disease of blood vessels and muscle, but in my case, as in millions of other cases, there are no easy answers. Pain is part of the disease.

If *The Path to Pain Control* had been on the shelf when I first reached out for help, I wouldn't have had to write it myself. Most published books on pain are written by medical experts, usually physicians or psychiatrists. Despite their good intentions, even books intended for the lay person seem to fall wide of the mark. The reason for this is reasonably simple. No one who has not personally experienced chronic pain can speak convincingly about how people in pain should cope. My own struggle taught me that we have an expertise that some experts don't. It has to do with being on the inside of the pain experience, being in our own skins. There's another crucial aspect to our expertise on pain. Because pain is best described as an interaction between a particular physical condition (yours) and a particular person (you), no two people's pain, no matter how similar their X rays or EKGs, can *feel* the same. Pain is a universal phenomenon, but it is uniquely filtered through each individual's nerves, body chemistry, and life experience. All the more reason why the key to pain control lies in your own hands, not with the medical experts. No one knows you better than you know yourself.

This is not to minimize the importance of medical and scientific expertise in dealing with chronic pain. As you will see, the chapters that follow reflect many of the latest developments in pain research. I am deeply committed to the notion that such knowledge should be accessible to all of us — we are, after all, those most immediately concerned — in terms we can understand. A number of physicians and researchers graciously shared their time and thinking with me precisely because they share my commitment to informed patient care.

■ ■ ■

Before going on to what *The Path to Pain Control* is all about, I want to backtrack a little to give a sense of how I moved — how slowly and with what resistance — from desperation to control and coping.

In the early stages of my illness the pain would come and go, building steadily for about ten days and then suddenly disappearing. When I was in pain I kept going, imagining that if I didn't give in, if I resisted, somehow or other the little devils that had invaded my body (note the medieval sense of anatomy) would get the message and move on. I had a doctor I greatly respected who kept telling me, "*You must be stronger than the pain.*" At the time I thought it was impressive advice. It certainly fit very neatly with my own world view of mind over matter, and personal and spiritual heroism.

But I think it's fair to say I got a little carried away. Even though the pain increased dramatically with walking, I walked relentlessly, determined to show "them" (and my own wavering sense of self) how strong I was. I even went on walks just for the sake of walking, setting out each time with renewed determination to outwalk the pain. As the pain mounted, I would grow more and more desperate. I was losing; *they* — the devils, the pain — were winning. Sometimes ten days would pass like that. Suddenly, just when I was at the depth of despair, the pain was gone. Relief and confusion. What had I done right? Had I finally beat the pain, or had it gone away of its own free will?

This confusion, which stems from the need to understand the comings and goings of pain, is one of the most typical problems experienced by people with chronic pain. We want to feel that we are in control and that we can do something concrete to combat this force that has invaded our bodies. The loss of control over our physical selves, over our mobility and our sanity (which is what is ultimately threatened) is a frightening thing. So we pit ourselves against pain, grit our teeth, try to block it out, play strong, sometimes even pretend to give in for a few days by taking to bed (but only pretend!). In short, we turn ourselves into emotional rubber bands in our attempts to outwit the Monster.

I had spent eighteen months riding the highs and lows of this dizzying roller coaster when two events occurred that were to have a decisive impact on my attitude toward pain. First, I met a Frenchwoman my own age who had multiple sclerosis. Along with other problems I didn't have, she had similar, though less severe, pain and cramping in her legs. She took one look at me limping from pillar to post, going out as many times a day as I could find excuses for, and kindly but firmly pointed out to me that I was manufacturing my pain — in other words, that I was a masochist. This had never occurred to me. In fact, it was such a threatening idea that I turned the accusation around, calling her a masochist for her self-limited walking. I felt she was overrestricting herself and giving in to being sick. But over time I began to see that while she was reaping the benefits of prudence, I was reaping the bitter fruit of my obstinately unrealistic attitude. I was in pain around the clock; she wasn't. Not that this was enough to convince me to change my habits, but it did open my eyes a crack.

Three months later, in December 1978, my pain pattern

suddenly changed. No more ten days on, ten days off. The pain went through the ceiling. Nothing seemed to stop it. The slightest walking, even standing up to cook, became excruciating. The painkillers I had carefully kept as a last resort (for when I *had* to capitulate) weren't strong enough. I started doubling the doses, cutting the "every four hours" to three, then two, and spent a good part of the month in bed. This time I had no choice; I was forced to listen. I had my first glimpse of real incapacity, which was terrifying. I also realized, for the first time, what it means to heed the body. I had to.

Shortly after this I returned to the United States from Europe, where I had been working as a freelance writer. I was scared and defeated. After a year and a half of trying to free myself from pain I was in more pain than ever. Instead of my outwitting pain, it had outwitted me. I had run through all the most powerful painkillers and was ready for morphine. I was in stalemate. On the brink of addiction, I realized it was time for me to take a closer look at my relationship to pain.

■ ■ ■

The doctor's words were simple enough: "You're just going to have to live with it. You're going to have to figure out how to live a very sedentary life." But their impact was devastating. Words I had dreaded; words I had never dreamt (only feared) would be said to me. Yet that physician finally brought me to my senses. The initial shock and disappointment (no cure, no end in sight?), the sense of outrage and injustice, gave way to a sense of relief. I had literally been waiting for someone else to tell me what my own body had been screaming for a year and a half. "You're just going to have to live with it." What's more, this was something I already knew, something so simple and so obvious that I had even gone so far as to announce to friends,

"If a doctor tells me it's not going to go away, *then* I'll really change my life." I was that conscious, if you can call it conscious, of my need for orders from higher up. And in my secular hierarchy, "higher up" meant "M.D."

Why was I so reluctant to listen to my own body? Primarily, I think, because to have done so would have been tantamount to surrender. It would have meant that I was doomed to stay sick. I was hell-bent on proving to myself and everyone who knew me that my life was unchanged as a result of my "problems with my health." I was a special breed: sick but invincible, despite all evidence to the contrary. So long as I had no guidelines, no rules, no medical answers, I could go on playing my own private game with pain — it can't get me down, I can take it, I'm a born coper — which meant that I could go on pretending that any day now the nightmare would be over. One morning I'd wake up feeling fine. But I knew all along I was pulling the wool over my eyes. My body had been through enough changes of climate, season, diet, activity, and inactivity to know that hot or cold, dry or humid, walking was Enemy Number One and that Healer Number One was rest. One thing chronic pain has taught me is that the body doesn't lie and that we can't lie to the body. It is the mind, not the body, that lets us lie to ourselves — but not for very long. Because mind and body are really one, the split can't last.

Ultimately the mind, like the body, demands honesty. This is the wonderful other side to the cruel experience of pain. We can go only so far with our carefully built defenses before they start springing leaks. When they do there is terror, confusion, depression, sometimes genuine breakdown. I know what a long, hard fight I put up to maintain my fragile edifice of pride, and I know how hard it was — and still is sometimes — to confront life without it. But in its place a whole new process was set in motion, a process of self-discovery that has not only enabled me to reduce my pain but also has immeasurably deepened and enriched my life. This process is what *The Path to Pain Control* is all about.

■ ■ ■

One of the first things I did after that shattering but ultimately sobering appointment with the neurologist was to go out and buy a small ruled notebook, on the cover of which I wrote "PAIN" in capital letters. Inside I began to record my reactions to pain, my fears, my dreams, my insights, my frustrations and anger, the thoughts and images that came to me at night when pain kept me awake. That journal launched me on the path to pain control.

I watched myself begin the old masochistic maneuvers. I began to notice my silent, passive way of manipulating attention from the people around me. My doctor's leveling with me had finally freed me to level with myself. At last I was able to admit that pain was something I had to come to terms with. Within a few short weeks of daily entries I realized that my pain journal had become more than an outlet for my long-held-in feelings: it had become the map of a new country I was finally ready to explore.

What I mean by a new country is a place — in this case a situation, chronic pain and my relationship to it — for which I, like most people, had little or no preparation. Most of us arrive in the land of pain alone, usually quite unexpectedly, often from one day to the next, like political refugees who have had to flee with nothing but the clothes on their backs. But unlike the refugee, who can sign up for a crash course in the language of his or her adopted country, we can take no crash courses in dealing with pain. Many of us manage to get by for weeks or months or even years pretending we are somewhere else. But sooner or later pain catches up with us, as it caught up with me, and we are forced to speak its language.

What is that language? First of all, it is a language of mind and body united. By taking your pain apart into its mind and body components and then reuniting them, *The Path to Pain Control* systematically explores both halves of the mind-body equation so that you will be able, as I have been, to reach the barest minimum of pain caused by your medical condition. As you begin to get a sense of what you bring to the experience of pain, you will be able to separate out the physical determinants of your pain from the personal ones. Along the way, you will pinpoint specific small changes you can make that will add up, over time, to significant pain reduction. Equally important, you will learn how to apply your best self — your strengths — to the process of coping.

The language of pain is also a language of multiplicity and possibility. It is a language of openness to new ideas and overlapping meanings. Pain is not simple, and our approach to it cannot be simple. Nor can it be single-minded. To meet pain's ever-changing challenge to our ingenuity, we need to cultivate a whole repertoire of skills — from the long-range, overall approaches that are developed in Chapters 3, 4, 5, 6, and 7 to the short-term, acute-episode techniques presented in the Pain Emergency Kit beginning on page 209.

I learned the hard way that pain cannot be killed. Expecting the impossible — total victory over pain — leads to overexertion, both mental and physical, and overexertion spells frustration, defeat, and usually more pain. It is only once you accept that you are not superman or superwoman, and that no one has the right to make you think you should be, that you will be on the path to pain control.

When this happens, you will feel yourself shifting gears. Pain will seem less like a hard-faced enemy and more like the life challenge it actually is. As you become aware of the many options you have — all the inner strengths you brought with you when you found yourself suddenly in the land of pain — you will feel yourself moving toward pain*less*ness, toward a more painless state of being. This is a learning process, a process that means reliance on self more than doctors, self more than pills, self more than a magic remedy you are waiting for "someone" to discover. Along the way you may find yourself, as I did, becoming involved in activities or kinds of thinking you might never have explored if pain hadn't entered your life.

As I write these words it is with a combination of hindsight (recognition of all the wrong turns I made along the way) and a growing sense that learning to live with pain is a continuous process. The path to pain control is a direction, an attitude, a way of looking at your life and at your pain that will lead you to feel less pain and to be better able to cope with the pain you do feel.

In the pages that follow, worked into the logical succession of chapters, you will find dozens of practical suggestions and ideas to help you extend your own repertoire of coping skills. As you read, be sure to keep in mind that everybody's pain is unique. There is no one trick or technique that will work for everyone, and even if you find something that seems to work for you, it may not *always* work. Because both pain and we are constantly changing, the key to coping is knowing that there are many, many different ways of dealing with it. Trial and error will show you which work best for you.

How to Use This Book

The Path to Pain Control is based on the assumption that you are willing to devote a few hours to the process of learning to cope more effectively with your pain. Its underlying purpose is twofold:

1. to show you how you can *reduce* your pain to a more manageable level, and
2. to help you devise a personal strategy for coping with the pain that remains.

This book is *not* a scientific treatise on the subject, nor does it discuss all the currently available treatments for pain. It is a step-by-step manual for sufferers — written by someone who knows the problems from the inside — to help you cope with the everyday issues that confront people with chronic pain. Ultimately, this book will work best for you if you use it as a guide to creating your own path to pain control.

The best way to use *The Path to Pain Control* is to read it straight through once. Don't worry about fully absorbing each exercise and integrating it into your life at first reading. It's more important to get a sense of the overall approach. (If you are in severe pain, you may want to begin with the Pain Emergency Kit on page 209.)

Once you have read the book in its entirety, go back and reread the sections that are most relevant to your personal situation. Feel free to pick and choose, adapting the ideas that fit your own requirements.

Certain chapters have been specifically designed to serve as reference sections to which you can return whenever the need arises. These include Chapters 9, 10, and 11, as well as the Pain Emergency Kit on pages 209–27 and the Coping Resource Guide on pages 231–42.

PART I

Paving
The Way

Where We Are Coming From

People with chronic pain spend most of their waking hours in a straitjacket no one else can see. We're hemmed in on all sides — by pain, by the fear of future pain and what will become of us, by the incredible number of calculations we have to make to get through each day (if I have to stand in line at the bank, will I be able to do the shopping; if I fix the broken screen door, will I be up to making dinner; if I do the laundry, what shape will I be in for the job interview tomorrow), by the pull to share our suffering with others and the pressure not to. On a typical day we're either in pain or dreading its return; either snowed from our last painkiller and sweating it out till the next one, or grimly trying to do without; and we're at work, whether it's out in the "world" or at home, where cleaning, shopping, cooking, and child care can easily make more than nine-to-five demands on our physical and mental resources. Through all the ups and downs of pain, no matter how dazed we are from Percodan or Valium or Darvon, our lives — with our work and our play, our friendships, loves, families, dreams, and aspirations — go on. Or do they? For some of us they do. For millions of others, chronic pain brings life itself to a halt.

Many of us no longer recognize ourselves after a year or two of pain. Our personalities have been shaken to the core, and what we most counted on — our close relationships, our marriages, our jobs — may well have fallen by the wayside. Our whole sense of life has radically changed since pain became a part of it, yet no one seems to understand our listlessness, our loss of hope, our lack of optimism. Other people can't *see* our pain, so how can they imagine what it's done to us? Only someone who has lived with chronic pain knows how insidious the process is. How subtly, over time, we learn to steel ourselves against each new attack, dulling ourselves to the sharp surprise of pain. Experience has taught us to expect the worst, because the worst keeps happening. It's a question of survival. But deep inside we know the price we've paid for this uneasy pact with pain: we mourn our old easygoing self, the pre-pain self who once naively thought all pain eventually went away.

The Invisible Millions

Multiply this tragic portrait by 40 million and you'll begin to have a sense of the staggering proportions of the pain problem in the United States alone. *Forty million people,* or one in six Americans, are in chronic pain. Put another way, there are enough men, women, and children in pain to fill seven of the nation's largest cities — New York, Los Angeles, Chicago, Philadelphia, Houston, Detroit, and Washington, D.C.

It is one of the ironies of the chronic pain experience that we can feel so alone when in fact we are part of a whole multitude of sufferers. Rheumatoid arthritis, one of the most painful types of arthritis, claims 6.5 million — and millions more suffer from other forms of the disease, including osteo-arthritis, ankylosing spondylitis, gout, and lupus, a serious systemic illness with between half a million and a million victims. Health authorities speak of 10 million Americans with recurrent migraines and 7 million with serious back problems. Facial pain from trigeminal neuralgia, myofascial syndrome, and temporomandibular joint syndrome is said to affect 8 million. The neurological and neuromuscular diseases such as Parkinson's, multiple sclerosis, and myasthenia gravis, all of which can cause pain, account for close to a million others. Two hereditary blood disorders, hemophilia and sickle-cell anemia, can cause severe pain to 25,000 and 50,000 respectively, the latter affecting primarily blacks. Shingles, difficult menstruation, and sports injuries are other leading causes of chronic pain. All this without counting the esti-mated 80,000 who sustain major injuries each year in industry, the 150,000 permanently disabled in automotive accidents, and the 2.5 million disabled veterans, more than 500,000 of them wounded in the Vietnam war.

When you add to these grim statistics the hundreds of thousands of newcomers who join our ranks each year, you can see why health writer Helen Neal has compared chronic pain to a full-scale epidemic and described it as one of the most serious problems on the nation's health agenda.

■ ■ ■

Where are all these people? They are everywhere — where you work, where you live, perhaps right in your own family. They are everywhere and they are nowhere, because pain is still a private, virtually taboo subject.

Based on my own experience and on the extensive, often extremely personal talks I had with each of the men and women I interviewed for this book, I am convinced that the devastating effects of chronic pain are, in great measure, the result of the way we have been conditioned to think about suffering. By keeping pain unmentionable, we have trapped ourselves in a set of punitive, moralistic attitudes that are tragically unsuited to the complex process of coping with chronic pain. As a result, people in pain remain locked in their separate suffering, unable to draw on each other's wisdom and experience. This conditioning can be reversed, but first we have to understand it.

The Model: Our Ideal Pain Behavior

Most Western countries, including our own, consider pain a miniature testing ground on which each of us gets the opportunity to be a hero or a heroine. According to this view, pain, like death, is one of those ultimate mysteries we are supposed to meet alone in a dark alley, courageously. And never talk about. We are not supposed to get help and not supposed to need it — except of course from pills, stoicism's silent partners. We are supposed to be strong and welcome the opportunity to suffer or, at the very least, to rise to the occasion without complaining. The rule of the day is Stiff Upper Lip, which is part and parcel of an unspoken code that tells us our pain should be unspoken too. What this really amounts to is a kind of censorship — unconsciously embedded in us all — that keeps pain in its place: invisible and silent.

All of us are part of this conspiracy of silence, whether or not we ourselves are in pain. Think how we fill with admiration when we learn that someone we see leading a full, active life is actually in constant pain — "but you'd never know." The fewer outward signs of pain there are (preferably none), and the worse we know or imagine it to be, the more admiration we tend to feel. Listen to some of the everyday expressions we use to show our approval of the "cover-up": "to suffer gracefully," "to bear it with dignity";

or, on the grimmer side, "to tough it out," "to bite the bullet." Now look at the facial expressions: the clenched jaw of the hero, the bead of sweat on the forehead, the fleeting grimace — all telltale signs of suppressed anguish. Many of these expressions are derived from war. *Vanquish, eliminate, attack:* this is the vocabulary — and macho model — with which we confront suffering. The expectation of soldierly valor in the face of pain is deeply rooted in our culture. Why else would we call the medicine we take to dull pain "painkillers"? We want and expect nothing short of lasting, total victory over pain. Of ourselves we expect nothing short of lasting, total heroism, day in and day out.

As long as we follow this model, like lemmings following each other off the edge of a cliff, we are doomed to make the same mistakes as those who have gone before us.

Coping with chronic pain is an art, and that art is what *The Path to Pain Control* is all about. Each of us, no matter what the cause of our pain, has the ability to transcend the mechanistic reaction our culture prescribes for pain. By recognizing the way our expectations not only keep us from coping but actually create more pain, we can learn to replace the negative model we have been taught with a positive, creative model that will allow each of us to reduce our pain to its lowest possible level and to cope with the pain that remains in the way best suited to our needs and personalities.

■ ■ ■

Pain isn't something we tend to think about before it happens to us, so when it strikes we do the most natural thing in the world: fall back on a powerful lifesaving instinct we probably didn't even know was there. The fight-or-flight response, as it is usually called, is an innate, autonomic survival mechanism that has probably been part of our physiological makeup for millions of years. When the slightest danger is perceived, this response automatically prepares the organism (in this case us) to fight for its life or flee. There is a rapid increase in the activity of the sympathetic nervous system, with a rise in blood pressure, faster breathing, and a heightened rate of metabolism and blood flow to the muscles of the arms and legs, the better to fight or flee with. Pain triggers fight-or-flight because it is perceived as a threat to survival.

When we are in pain, this instinctive reaction is accompanied by an overlay of more sophisticated behavior that may initially make sense but that eventually beats us at our own game. Each of us has our own variation on the prevailing cultural pattern.

My own response in the early weeks of pain is a good example. When I first got sick and was living in Europe, I was extremely frightened. Although never an athletic type, I had lived twenty-seven years as a fairly active human being. From one day to the next I found myself weak in the knees; then, in the course of a few short days, I was walking as if I were drunk. Shortly after that the aches I had been experiencing became severe pain. With my doctor's encouragement I kept going in spite of the pain. I was determined to fight. I walked obsessively. I guess in the back of my mind I was waiting for the second-wind phenomenon I'd heard about from my runner friends, hoping that if I kept at it long enough I'd eventually shake whatever had me by the legs and break into an elegant trot. My heroics failed to do the trick. What I eventually broke into was pure pain and a two-week stay in the hospital.

Many of us spend years playing subtle variations on our original crisis pattern because we can't accept that there's something fundamentally wrong with the whole approach. We blame ourselves instead of an ideology that's guaranteed to lead to feelings of inadequacy, frustration, and despair. In the name of willpower and determination, or mind over matter, we're fighting so hard that we lose sight of a very crucial distinction, the distinction between acute and chronic pain. As a result we get stuck in patterns of behavior derived from the fight-or-flight response long after they have ceased to be appropriate. We keep punching long after our opponent has left the ring.

Acute vs. Chronic Pain

All pain can be excruciating, blinding, terrifying. But the saving grace of acute pain — the pain of a broken nose, the pain that follows open-heart surgery, even the pain of a bad burn — is that you know it is going to go away. Usually each day is a little better than the day before, so that even when the pain is intense you know you are on the mend. Chronic pain is different. By definition it exists over time (*chronos* being the ancient Greek word for "time"). Unlike acute pain, chronic pain is not part of a healing process. Just the opposite is often true, as with arthritis, for example, where the pain is a sign of active disease or of its crippling consequences. Acute pain serves the positive purpose of warning you of an immediate danger; chronic pain often seems to have no discernible meaning. Another distinguishing feature of chronic, as opposed to acute, pain is its unpredictability and intermittency. Most people with chronic pain are not in pain twenty-four hours a day. Rather, we are often in pain and rarely know when to expect a letup or a recurrence. It is this episodic aspect of chronic pain that most people find so hard to take.

Our cultural model is geared to meet (at best) the needs of acute pain, which is a crisis situation. Chronic pain, however frightening and demanding it may be, is *not* a crisis situation. It only seems like one. When your house is burning down, you grab the baby and run out the door. When you're in chronic pain, you can't keep reacting as if your life were a house afire. But we do — millions of us. Why?

There are several answers. First of all, we don't know any other response. Nothing in our past experience has prepared us for chronic pain. All that most of us have to go on is our childhood training in scraped knees and playground fights, or the occasional broken limb or impacted wisdom tooth, and that doesn't seem to stand us in very good stead. What we learned as children ("Boys don't cry," "Now be a big girl") is deeply ingrained by the time we're adults, thanks to years of reinforcement from doctors, dentists, teachers, parents, and tough-skinned Hollywood cowboys. Second, there's a time factor. You don't know ahead of time that you're going to have chronic pain. You *think* you have acute pain — at first you do — so you react the way you've learned to react to acute pain. Only over time, very gradually, do you begin to realize that the pain you've been expecting to disappear has in fact become chronic. By the time that realization dawns, you may have spent months or even years without a long-term strategy for coping, because you optimistically — or stubbornly — believed you wouldn't need one.

There's a third reason. Fear. Despite the fact that the overwhelming majority of us will experience physical suffering at some point in our lives, in our pill-oriented, high-med-tech culture we have come to expect that pain need not and should not occur. Like some strange mistake, some aberration of nature, it can be magically erased by aspirin or, if we get really desperate, "killed" by one of the superdrugs like Demerol or morphine. We don't want to believe that there's pain that outlasts even these powerful agents.

Our fear of protracted suffering looms so large that we do everything in our power to bring pain down to size. If you think about it, one way we can control (or *think* we can control) chronic pain is by treating it as if it were acute.

It's our way of not recognizing chronic pain, not granting it legitimacy in our lives, just as some nations don't recognize each other's governments. Treat it as acute and it will go away. The underlying assumption here is that if you admit for one second that your pain is chronic, it will *never* go away. There's an element of superstition here too, a trace of the curiously medieval thinking that often takes over when we moderns are afraid. We tend to personify our pain as a monster, a dictator, a devil, or some other awful creature. Secretly we believe we're involved in a battle of wills: if we can just be tough enough or virtuous enough long enough, the malevolent being that has invaded our body will eventually get the message and throw in the sponge.

The Consequences

These strategies are clever, but they rarely succeed. Heroism is fine when it works, but when your own self-image is at stake, as it is with chronic pain, the risks are high indeed. As anyone with chronic pain knows all too well, the tough-it-out-alone attitude takes a heavy toll on its practitioners. Keeping a stiff upper lip while a tooth is being pulled or a broken arm is being set is one thing, but no one can go on being heroic day after day. It takes a lot of energy to keep retrieving the image of the hero you think you're supposed to be. Study after study has shown that people who try to fight their pain end up in more pain than ever because of the stress involved. And when the brave front crumbles, as sooner or later it must, the self behind the mask crumbles too, into feelings of despair and anger that often spill over onto those around us.

Everyone knows what happens to a kettle when the water starts to boil: it screams or, in more whimsical parlance, "whistles." Letting off steam is a natural, healthy, and —

for a kettle — inevitable response to pressure. Being in a lot of pain and having to be tough and heroic day after day means you have no way of letting off steam. You're a kettle without a spout. What happens? You turn it inward, and you do what everyone else does: let it off anyway, in all sorts of little ways. It's just as inevitable for you as it is for a kettle. You get tense, irritable, and angry; yell at your kids, your spouse, your lover, or your best friend; pick a fight with a sales clerk or a bus driver — in short, you take it out on anyone who has the misfortune to be in your way. Not only does this end up hurting everyone around you but, as we'll see farther on, all those negative emotions can have a very adverse effect on your health. And on your pain.

Replacing the Model

We have inherited a model for coping with pain that clearly does more harm than good. Even at its best, it can't lead to pain control, because when you substitute heroism for insight, all your energy gets channeled into *taking* pain instead of reducing it. Whether or not we adhere to the model, it takes an awesome toll on our psyches and our bodies. Those of us who fit the pattern pay a mercilessly high price for coping so "well," while those who can't sustain the rigorous stoicism that's held up for approval are punished by feelings of failure and despair. Whether the short run registers success or failure, in the long run both success and failure translate into physical and emotional stress and are recycled into pain, creating a self-perpetuating circle of suffering. The model is faulty; it must be replaced.

Because it is so different from acute pain in its relationship to time, chronic pain calls for a whole different plan of action. You already possess the ability to develop a pain strategy that's tailor-made to your own needs and aspirations and medical situation. Based on self-knowledge and a careful analysis of the crucial factors that make your pain function, it is the most powerful tool you have for pain control. Most amazing of all, the more you use it the more you will have it. But there is nothing magical or mystical about your ability to control your own pain. The latest, most exciting developments in science suggest that the inner resources you will learn to mobilize through the techniques presented in this book translate into physiological processes that can actually break the hold of chronic pain.

2

Toward a More Painless State of Being

Almost everyone with long-standing pain has been to see at least one doctor. Most of us have been through a whole series. Typically, we've been in and out of several hospitals and have been tested, scrutinized, and stamped "seen" by more than a dozen certified physicians. Yet our pain often eludes the best of doctors and the best of treatments. With all the scientific breakthroughs we have seen in our lifetimes, pain is still one of the most tantalizing and most tenacious of medical mysteries. People in pain get passed from hand to hand, from specialist to specialist, faster than hot potatoes. It's not hard to understand why.

Chronic pain is the supreme insult to today's physicians, who have at their fingertips an array of technical equipment no less impressive than the galaxy of dials an astronaut commands. The comparison is not haphazard: doctors and patients alike expect medicine to navigate the inner reaches of the human body with the same astonishing success our astronauts have shown in navigating outer space. Given the

14

unprecedented strides medicine has made during the past hundred and fifty years, it's not surprising that we expect so much from doctors and that doctors expect so much from themselves. Ever since epidemiologists began identifying specific bacilli in the nineteenth century, one by one such devastating diseases as malaria, typhoid, polio, and diphtheria have all but disappeared from the "developed" world. With each of these medical triumphs it has become increasingly seductive to think of the body as a territory to be known and conquered, with physicians as the conquerors. Since 1885, when Pasteur successfully treated a small boy with antirabies vaccine, victory has been added to victory. No wonder science has become a secular religion, with doctors replacing priests in the popular imagination: they have, after all, performed the most visible miracles.

Why is it, then, that with all these advances, doctors are still in such a quandary when it comes to chronic pain? In part because pain research has proceeded along the same mechanistic lines as most other medical research: by pursuing a single cause, a single guilty germ or missing gene or damaged nerve, when it is now known that pain, like all bodily processes, is produced and contoured by many distinct, converging forces. Pain treatment has largely taken its cues from pain research, with new "modalities" and new machines following swiftly on the heels of each new scientific theory. Specific treatments such as transcutaneous nerve stimulation (TNS), dorsal column stimulation (DCS), nerve blocks, and more radical surgical procedures such as sympathectomy, rhizotomy, and chordotomy may initially provide relief for a certain percentage of people, but because these treatments focus on a single system, their long-term effectiveness is less impressive. Pain, like blood, often finds new routes, even when a major pathway has been blocked or severed.

■ ■ ■

It's not easy to step back from your own pain and look at it philosophically, especially when you're in the midst of an intense bout. But I think it's clear to all of us who have experienced chronic pain that pain is more than just an unpleasant sensation or, as the pros put it, a "noxious stimulus." Because it is felt in the body and suffered in the mind, pain straddles the two worlds that science has been battling for centuries to keep apart. By its very nature it seems to make a mockery of the rationalistic, lock-and-key orientation that has characterized Western medicine ever since Descartes. *We* know that pain echoes deep within us, evoking a primal connection of mind and body that goes back before the advent of Western civilization. That resonance of the physical on the psyche (and vice versa) is what makes pain so difficult to bear. Paradoxically, it is also a source of hope. Because mind and body interact to create pain, *you* have the potential to control your pain more effectively than any doctor. No matter how well trained or well intentioned a physician is, no doctor has ever spent a sleepless night in your body, and neither your doctor nor your closest friends can ever know how deeply pain has cut into your life. No one knows you, body and soul, better than you know yourself.

How Much Is How Bad?

There are all kinds of theories about how pain messages travel through the body, and all sorts of techniques for measuring the exact fraction of a second when pain volunteers first detect the sensation of pain from a "noxious stimulus." But because most research on pain takes place in laboratories far removed from actual human suffering, even fellow researchers have questioned the usefulness of some of the results. By studying how much pain healthy male college students can take for three dollars an hour, or under what conditions electrically shocked rats do *not* scream, researchers do not necessarily arrive at data relevant to the experience of people in chronic pain. The problem with so much current research is that it quantifies pain. How much does it hurt? How bad is your arthritis? That doesn't tell you what to do about pain.

Dr. James Hardy of the University of Pennsylvania and Dr. Harold Wolff of Cornell University recently created a 10-point scale to measure pain intensity. Arthritis pain received the lowest score, 1, while a cigarette burn was classed as 10. Whatever scientific validity this sort of work may have, such abstract, clinical measurements of pain are irrelevant to people experiencing real-life, protracted pain. What you make of the experience of pain and how it affects you in your daily and ongoing life is something that can't be measured on a universal scale or abstracted into a theory.

What *we* are after in *The Path to Pain Control* is not quantity but quality: how you feel as a person in the midst of pain, how your pain feels to you, and what you can do to bring it down to a more tolerable level more of the time.

The Exciting Possibilities of Mind-Body Research

Encompassing as it does the double face of mind and body, pain has been likened to Janus, the Roman god of doors, whose twin faces looked forward and backward at the same time. Yet mind and body are not two faces looking in opposite directions; they are one — a single, united being in which the emotions and physical events interact in a still largely unfathomed way. Some of the most promising medical research on pain is now zeroing in on this multifaceted interaction. A number of researchers, including Dr. Ronald Melzack, one of the foremost authorities on pain and author of

The Puzzle of Pain, believe that such factors as a person's past experience of pain, belief system, and hopes and fears for the future all play a role in determining, in Dr. Melzack's words, "the actual pattern of nerve impulses that ascend from the body to the brain itself. In this way, pain becomes a function of the whole individual."

There is already sufficient evidence to show that the mind can and does alter the body's experience of pain. The classic study on this theme was published in 1946 by the late Harvard anesthesiologist Henry K. Beecher, who was a field doctor on the Anzio beachhead during World War II. Observing the behavior of severely wounded soldiers as they were brought in from battle, Beecher was astonished to find that only one man in three accepted morphine when it was offered. When he returned to clinical practice after the war, Beecher offered morphine to civilians who had been hospitalized for injuries similar to those the soldiers had sustained. Four out of five accepted, saying that their pain was severe. Beecher's evaluation of his findings showed that the soldiers at Anzio had not lost the ability to *feel* pain; the decisive factor, he hypothesized, was their euphoria at being released from combat. Their terrible wounds were a cause of relief and gratitude, whereas the civilians' similar injuries, unexpected and frightening, constituted a serious disruption in the natural flow of their lives. Beecher concluded that the difference in the need for morphine between the two groups could be accounted for only by their different attitudes toward being injured.

Another study, in the early 1960s, tested the pain tolerance of an American nurse who had spent ten years among the Eskimo in Alaska. Immediately after her return to her home state, her tolerance was found to be extremely high for an American; it was, in fact, as high as that of the Eskimo among whom she had lived, a group noted worldwide for its unusually high pain tolerance. Retested a mere six months later, the nurse's tolerance had returned to the expected norm for an American. The ability to withstand severe pain, the New York University investigators concluded, must be due to cultural attitudes; what's more, this study suggests, such attitudes can be acquired — and lost — within relatively short periods of time.

One woman I interviewed had previously had a mastectomy. When she was hospitalized again four years later, she was afraid that her pain was due to a recurrence of cancer. Given her breast-cancer history, this was not an unreasonable fear, and it was shared by her doctor. Only when the bone scan came back negative was she transformed, suddenly, into a very relieved lower-back patient. The pain was still there, but its dragonesque proportions had vanished. Many people have experienced similar relief on learning that their cluster headaches are just that: cluster headaches and not brain tumors. The pain may not always disappear, but it does diminish. Emotional relief actual *becomes* physical relief.

The Implications for Chronic Pain

If beliefs or attitudes can dramatically alter our experience of pain, perhaps we can learn to weed out or eliminate those states of mind that enhance pain, and cultivate the kinds of thinking and activities that reduce it. This hypothesis is behind the current wave of interest in the so-called "placebo effect."

Physicians and pharmacologists have long been fascinated by the fact that a consistent percentage — hovering around 35 percent — of patients who receive a placebo (the proverbial sugar pill) instead of a pharmacologically active drug exhibit physical reactions consistent with the characteristic results of the drug they *believe* they have received.

In the early 1960s a group of medical students at Albert Einstein College of Medicine in New York City took part in an experiment in which they were told they would be given either a stimulant or a sedative, in order to test the effectiveness of each. They were given detailed information about the effects of each drug, including possible adverse reactions. Actually, both "drugs" were placebos. The results were dramatic. More than half the students experienced reactions typical for each supposed medication; those who thought they had received a sedative went back to their rooms and fell asleep, while those who thought they had been given stimulants became agitated and hyper-alert. Adverse side effects included dizziness, gastrointestinal irritation, and runny eyes. In a study of arthritis patients, when a placebo pill was substituted for aspirin or cortisone, the number of people reporting improvement from the placebo was equal to that responding to the two conventional antiarthritics.

In a fascinating article published in the *New England Journal of Medicine* in 1979, Dr. Herbert Benson pointed out that while every remedy for angina introduced over the past two hundred years was effective in 70 to 90 percent of patients when first administered, as soon as it was superseded by another therapy the effectiveness of the earlier treatment dropped to 30 or 40 percent. According to Dr. Benson, only the doctor's belief in the value of each new treatment and the patient's belief in the doctor could account for the first-time success of so many different remedies. Actually, the patient's belief in a treatment's chance of working is part of every doctor's bag of tricks. It is an old truism of medicine that doctors "should treat as many patients as possible with the new drugs while they still have the power to heal."

The placebo effect has also been demonstrated in a number of nondrug techniques, including acupuncture, X ray, surgery that was not performed although the patient was told it had been, as well as with transcutaneous nerve stimulation. What all these studies show is that the power of suggestion — a product of the recipient's trust in the person administering the treatment, as well as the latter's belief in the treatment — can have powerful physiological results. Additional studies have established that the stronger the suggestion, and the greater the subject's need to believe it, the more likely a placebo effect is to take place.

Originally it was thought that only ignorant, highly gullible people responded to placebos, and placebo responders were ridiculed for being "conned" into thinking they had actually been helped. It is now known that almost everyone can respond to a placebo under the proper conditions, and that even our response to active drugs, such as aspirin or penicillin, partakes of the placebo effect. Rather than being a dummy effect, as was previously believed, a number of investigators are now suggesting that the placebo's ability to relieve pain may quite literally be due to the power of suggestion. According to the results of an experiment with dental patients reported in the British medical journal *Lancet* (September 1978), belief in a placebo may mobilize the release of the body's own pain relievers, or *endorphins.*

Endorphins: The Morphine Within

Identified almost simultaneously in 1973 by research teams in Scotland and the United States, endorphins are naturally occurring brain enzymes that are almost identical to morphine in chemical structure and behavior. Both endorphins and morphine produce pain relief by binding to specific receptor sites in the brain. But unlike morphine, which is a powerful, potentially addicting drug with serious side effects, endorphins are part of the body's innate healing system. Their discovery has generated a climate of great optimism among pain researchers.

Dr. Jon D. Levine, Dr. Newton C. Gordon, and Dr. Howard L. Fields, authors of the *Lancet* article, made history with their discovery that naloxone, a drug known to reverse the effects of morphine, also reversed the pain relief produced by a placebo in dental patients studied at the University of California Medical Center in San Francisco. No morphine was actually given in the course of the experiment, but those patients who *believed* they had been given morphine experienced an increase in pain after taking naloxone. The scientists' conclusion? That endorphins, morphine's doubles, must be involved in the placebo response.

At first endorphins were likened to morphine; it now appears that morphine may be only a pale shadow of the powerful internal painkillers we all possess. Recent work in California has disclosed the existence of a brain chemical two hundred times more powerful than morphine. The Stanford University researchers named their 1979 discovery "dynorphin" (from the Greek *dynamis* — "power" — and from *endorphin*). So far, scientists aren't sure exactly what distinguishes dynorphin from its less powerful but no less astonishing siblings. "With something as powerful as this," says Dr. Avram Goldstein, head of the group that made the discovery, "you can't doubt that it has a significant function. Now the problem is to find out what that function is."

The existence of morphine-like substances within the brain itself, and thus within each one of us, has raised the hope that internal substances for pain relief will eventually replace external ones. Because endorphins ("the morphine within") are concentrated in the region of the brain known as the limbic system — the so-called "old" brain that is particularly involved with strong emotions — endorphin research is proceeding into exciting terrain indeed. If belief, suggestion, and other powerful emotional states (perhaps including laughter*) can trigger a placebo response, and if, as the *Lancet* article suggests, the placebo effect mobilizes endorphins, we may well be moving toward a new integration of mind and body in the treatment of pain.

Putting It All Together

By studying the conditions under which the placebo effect takes place, scientists hope to understand the specific processes that govern the mind-body relationship. The work on endorphins dovetails with research currently under way at Harvard, where Dr. Herbert Benson and his co-workers are engaged in a study of a number of non-Western healing practices such as yoga, meditation, and ritual breathing. "We hope to learn to what extent a thought process can alter physiology in definable, reproducible ways," Benson explains. "By observing the extreme in advanced religious practitioners, we will know the limits of possibility."

I discussed this research with Dr. Joan Borysenko, instructor in medicine at Harvard, where she is a member of Benson's team. If the promising leads she described to me are supported by future study, scientists may soon be able to explain the distinct physiological makeup of emotional states such as hope, fear, and anxiety, and their impact on the human organism. The results of studies by

* In *Anatomy of an Illness,* Norman Cousins describes the self-prescribed laughter treatment that he credits with helping to bring about his dramatic recovery from a crippling collagen disease. Cousins explores the possibility that the unorthodox treatment he pursued, which also included massive doses of intravenous vitamin C, may have been a "mammoth venture in self-administered placebos." Such a hypothesis, he continues, "bothers me not at all. Respectable names in the history of medicine, like Paracelsus, Holmes, and Osler, have suggested that the history of medication is far more the history of the placebo effect than of intrinsically valuable and relevant drugs."

Benson's group and other researchers already show that various techniques can lead to a physiological response that is the exact opposite of fight-or-flight. This state of inner calm, which has been termed the "relaxation response," appears to be every bit as much a part of our instinctive survival apparatus as the fight-or-flight response; what's more, it can be cultivated and induced at will. If the scientists are right, they will be documenting for the first time in the history of Western medicine what the sages of the East have known for millennia: that the mind has extraordinary powers to transform the life of the body.

■ ■ ■

This book proceeds on the assumption that when we have learned to use our minds to their fullest pain-reducing capacities we will have learned, as Norman Cousins did, that the placebo itself is no longer necessary. Placebo effects don't have to take place in laboratories; and since a placebo doesn't have to be a pill, a whole range of activities can, with the proper attitude, be channeled into a personal strategy for pain control. When all is said and done, the placebo, in Cousins's words, is "only a tangible object made essential in an age that feels uncomfortable with intangibles." What the placebo makes tangible is belief, our own belief in a more painless state of being. *The Path to Pain Control* has been designed to guide you, step by step, toward that state.

PART II

The Path
to
Pain Control

3

Chronic Redefined: Claiming Your Pain in Your Own Terms

Most of us, as we've already seen, do not create our own response to pain. We inherit it. This is where the trouble begins. The prevailing Western model, a sophisticated up-date of the fight-or-flight response, preaches a heroism whose only approved "out" is drugs — painkillers. When a large part of your energy goes into fighting your pain, blocking it out, pushing it under, or any of a dozen other common strategies for pretending it isn't there, you're both in pain and in flight from pain. Your best energy gets taken up in minute-to-minute survival tactics that are ill suited to the nuanced, ever-changing, highly personal experience of chronic pain. The net effect of all these variations on the fight-or-flight theme is to lock you into a vestigial response that immobilizes your potential for coping just when you need it most.

The Way Out

To move beyond this no-win fight with pain, you need to replace instinct with ingenuity and insight. The first step on the path to pain control is learning to stay right where you are, stop fighting invisible mastodons, and take a good, calm look around. Chronic pain, when you stand still long enough to catch your breath, is not the monster it's cracked up to be.

Part of the problem comes from the word *chronic* itself, which takes us to the very edge of fear. There we stop, teetering on the brink, afraid to look ahead yet unable to go back to where we were. Before we can learn to cope with chronic pain we need to cope with the word *chronic*.

Chronic Redefined

For most of us, *chronic* conjures up a terrible image somewhere in the back of our minds. For me it was a steel door slamming shut and the sound of a key irrevocably turning in the lock. *Chronic* meant "doomed for life." All *chronic* really means is "of or relating to time." Chronic pain is pain that has a relationship to time. How *much* time is not the real issue. The real issue, whether your pain lasts six months or six years, is how your chronic pain feels to you and what you make of the experience once you have reduced your pain to its lowest possible level.

Pain as a Learning Process

Living with pain may well be the most challenging experience you've had to face in your whole life. It is for many people; it certainly was for me. There are no ready-made solutions. If there were, word would have gotten out long ago and we would all now know the answer. We have that old paradox to ponder: "No man is an island." No one is alone, yet because each person's pain has a unique history both in its medical origin and in relation to the particular human being in whom the physical situation unfolds, each of us has to find and follow our own path to pain control.

Still, we can share a great deal with one another. One of the first people I spoke with about pain described it as a "learning process." From Valerie, whose rheumatoid arthritis was quite severe, I learned to think of pain itself as a teacher. "If you are open to learning," she said, "your pain will tell you exactly how to cope." I found her words to be absolutely true, once I began to *unlearn* the negative strategies I had latched on to in my first year and a half of pain. Much of life's best learning depends on just this sort of unlearning, or freeing of the mind.

Being in the Here and Now

As we've already seen, there has been a great deal of cultural brainwashing about pain. In recent years, television and the other mass media have only made matters worse. In a typical evening's programming, we are treated to a strange collage of contradictory images. On the one hand, we see hero after hero endure unimaginable suffering with unflinching toughness. On the flip side of the coin, every twelve minutes, whimpering sufferers of "mild discomfort" reach gratefully for the bottle with "more pain reliever."

Our Western pain ideology is particularly damaging because it keeps us in a state of denial about what is really happening to us. Our energy gets spent in sustaining a grand illusion of coping when in fact all we have learned — at best — is how to push pain away for a few minutes at a time. With chronic pain, that is not enough. So long as we are always "elsewhere" in our minds, we deprive ourselves of the possibility of moving toward a more painless state of being.

Genuine pain control comes from being grounded in the here and now — knowing where you are, surveying the terrain with a sense of adventure, and claiming your reality in your own terms. In this chapter and the four that follow, we will take this process step by step, so that by the end of Chapter 7, "Turning Pain Energy into Life Energy," you will have acquired a thorough mastery of what makes your pain unique, learned concrete ways of reducing it to its lowest possible level, and mapped out your own strategy for coping with the pain that remains.

The process begins with an exploration of that "place" we all unconsciously refer to when we say we are "in pain."

This Place Called Pain

Sometimes pain is so overwhelming, so engulfing, that it almost seems to be outside us. It's as if the world itself had turned into pain. If you think about it, we come to this spatial view of pain quite naturally. It's built into our thinking when we say something as clear-cut and straightforward as "I'm in pain." We don't say, "Pain is in me." This expression does not reflect the scientific view of pain, since we all know rationally that pain is inside us, and not the other way around. Rather, it reflects the larger-than-life dimension of pain in our imagination.

We didn't choose to enter this place called pain. Most of us were either catapulted into it by a sudden injury or else gradually took up residence through the slower process of disease. In either case, however we acquired our "onerous citizenship," as Susan Sontag calls it, physical suffering was our passport. That's what got us here. But what does *here* really mean? What does it look like? What greets us when we arrive?

The place is littered with the words of past inhabitants

who overdramatize the whole experience and overwhelm us with the sense that somehow we just aren't living it on a high enough plane. Great writers have glorified the experience of pain as a stepping-stone to enhanced sensitivity. Ralph Waldo Emerson declared: "He has seen but half the universe who never has been shown the house of pain." And Dante Alighieri wrote: "The more perfect the thing, the more deeply it feels pleasure, and also pain." Perhaps most dangerous of all, because they come from people we love and trust, are the well-meant encouragements of friends and acquaintances who've never experienced chronic pain themselves. Their comments are usually clichés, most of which paint pain in emotionally stultifying and stunting colors Typically, they range from deep purple ("Oh, you *poor* thing," "You're so *brave,*" "I'm so sorry") to scarlet ("You really are amazing, the way you handle it," "I think your pain has deepened you") to beatific blue ("She's never looked more beautiful"), treating pain as a means to spiritual grace. As a person with chronic pain you have not only the right but the need to question every single one of these interpretations. No matter how well intentioned, all these hand-me-down views of chronic pain are chronically unhealthy.

Claiming the Place Called Pain for Yourself

Inherited interpretations don't give you a chance to figure matters out for yourself. They also function as a subtle form of suggestion. If you believe that pain is doing wonders for your character, you have an investment in its continuation. As John, a thirty-two-year-old disabled Vietnam veteran pointed out, even our everyday response to trivial health matters has a tendency to encourage feelings of sickness:

> "Someone will sneeze. The other person will say, "Bless you!" Someone else will say, "Have you got a cold?"

This is a suggestion to the person who sneezed who has either to negate it or else to have a cold! Nine times out of ten the person walks in the next day with a cold."

In addition, inherited interpretations sugarcoat the experience of chronic pain. They encourage you to deny or repress the very real feelings of resentment, fear, and anger that everybody feels when faced with this protracted challenge to his or her physical and mental well-being.

In order to reduce your pain to its lowest possible level and cope most successfully with the pain that remains, you need to be directly in touch with *all* your reactions, including those that society does not reward with expressions of approval and admiration. When you don't know what you're really feeling, you can't learn from your experience and move on. Interpretations, whether positive or negative, filter your experience through other people's eyes. Learning to see your pain as *you* see it, not as someone else does or as someone else says you should see it, is a major step on the path to pain control. By claiming the place called pain for yourself you can take the "sting" out of chronic pain and free your best energy for coping.

Cleaning House

The mind can interpret pain in a way that lessens it, but because of our conditioning, the mind's interpretation more often increases pain. Whether we make bearing pain heroic or virtuous or dignified or a means of redemption, we're adding to our pain, filling it with meaning when we should be keeping it empty. The Zen teacher Shunryu Suzuki advocated a periodic "general housecleaning of your mind." "You may want many things . . . but before you put something in your room, it is necessary for you to take out something. If you do not, your room will become crowded with old, useless junk." When you're in chronic pain it's difficult to find the clarity of mind that will let you see through the clutter of interpretations that have accumulated over time. This is why the concept of *recognition* is so important.

What Is Recognition?

Recognition is the knowledge that comes from experience and observation *together*. In dealing with chronic pain, recognition is essential because only when you really know and understand your pain will you have the ability to change it. Recognition is more than just looking at something and saying "I see it." Before you can recognize something, you have to know all about it, know its stamp and contour the way you know the back of your own hand. Recognition gives you a place to move *out* of: when you don't know where you are, you're really stuck. As you go through the sequence of exercises in the next few pages, recognition will become more than an idea. It will become a skill.

The Plain Ordinary Pain Scale

Abstract measurements of pain such as the one cited in Chapter 2 aren't much use when it comes to chronic pain, but a scale of your own that allows you to keep track of the fluctuations in your pain can be an important tool for pain control. When *you* determine how much is how bad, the measurements are meaningful indicators. You begin to recognize the situations and treatments that reduce your pain and those that increase them. As you proceed on the path to pain control, you'll want to refer to the measurements you make right now as a base line for control.

On a scale of 1 to 10, where 10 is the worst pain you can

imagine and 1 is the least amount of pain you've ever felt (not counting 0), record your personal pain levels for the following: your pain level right now while you are reading these words; the worst pain you ever personally experienced; and the level of pain you most frequently have when you have pain. If your pain comes and goes, try to pinpoint the intensity it most often has. Place an X at the appropriate place on the scale for each category. If your pain level falls between two numbers, place your X where you feel it belongs.

Pain Level	Today's Date _____									
Right Now	1	2	3	4	5	6	7	8	9	10
Worst I Ever Felt	1	2	3	4	5	6	7	8	9	10
Most Frequent Level	1	2	3	4	5	6	7	8	9	10

Grounded Theory

Sociologists Barney Glaser and Anselm Strauss of the Medical Sociology Department at the University of California Medical Center in San Francisco have developed a fascinating concept they call Grounded Theory. According to them, in order to get an inside view of any area of human life, an investigator's first impressions must be constantly reworked and taken back into the "field" to be checked and verified. Instead of inventing a theory or interpretation and then looking at your subject, first you study the subject and make your theory from the ground up. That way theories are never abstract. Grounded theory is theory with its feet on the ground, theory that's rooted in experience.

In an investigation of chronic pain, the field, for each of us, is our own pain experience. In the following pages you will join six other people in pain on an exploration of what the place called pain feels like to you. Each of the self-portraits below looks at one facet, or aspect, of your pain experience. I have found this the quickest and most revealing way to free the mind from its old ways of responding to pain.

Self-Portrait 1

Self-Portrait 1 is a simple introduction: name, age, reason for pain, occupation. After reading the first six self-portraits, add your own in the space provided at the bottom.

My name is Rosalie. I'm twenty-six years old. A year and a half ago I was in a car crash on the way home from a trip with a guy I had just decided to break up with. Since the accident I've been in a back brace, and the pain in my back radiates into my legs. I work nine to five as a receptionist, but my true love is art.

My name is Paul. I'm thirty-five years old. I had a herniated disk two years ago, followed by a laminectomy and a spinal fusion. Now it feels like the whole thing is starting up again, only a little farther down. The pain is mainly in my lower and middle back. I used to do carpentry, but since I've had back trouble I've been doing general contracting.

My name is Edna. I'm forty-three years old. I worked in a textile factory until I was hurt on the job five years ago by a loading crane. Besides the pain in my back, neck, and legs I have terrible abdominal pains as a result of a perforated ulcer I got after the accident. I haven't been able to find work since I got out of the hospital.

My name is Frank. I'm fifty-two years old. I've been in pain ever since I can remember. I had osteomyelitis when I was five, which left me with one short leg and very little mobility in my left arm. I also have arthritis in the knees, hips, and hands. I work full time as a psychologist in an inner-city school system.

My name is Jack. I'm sixty years old. I've been in pain on and off since World War Two, when I was wounded in the leg. I was in a car accident fifteen years ago. As a result I developed posttraumatic gout that affects my legs, hands, and feet. I work full time as the director of research for a major trade publication.

My name is Hannah. I'm seventy-four years old. I've had rheumatoid arthritis for the past thirty-five years. The pain started in my neck, but over the years it's spread to my hips, my shoulders, my elbows, and my knees. I was very active until about two years ago but now I can barely walk around my own apartment.

Self-Portrait 2: The 10 A.M. News

In Self-Portrait 2, you're going to use the concept of *recognition* to obtain a very simple, straightforward report on your pain at 10 A.M. on a typical weekday. Where are you? What are you doing? In the box provided, record the level of pain you usually feel in that place and at that time of day, based on the Plain Ordinary Pain Scale on page 34. Tell where in your body the pain is, and describe it succinctly and "objectively," as if you were a journalist. If you rarely have pain under the circumstances you've described, record that you are not in pain. First read the other portraits; then enter your own.

Rosalie   5

I'm at work. I'm sitting at the front desk working the switchboard. The mornings are very hectic here because we get a lot of orders. Between nine and one I'm almost constantly on the phone with customers. A lot of people also come in and I'm the one to greet them. My pain is moderate to strong. My back and my left leg are throbbing.

Paul   0

I'm in a building where my partner and I are designing a showroom for a sportswear manufacturer. I'm sitting on a stool at a drafting table examining the plans with the president of the firm. My back is stiff and achy but I wouldn't really call it painful.

Edna   10

I'm at the kitchen table having coffee. Every morning I make breakfast for my husband, but after he leaves for work I'm alone in the house. Since I lost my job I really haven't had anything to do. The TV is in the kitchen, so I don't have to go back upstairs. The pains in my stomach are awful; my arms and legs are throbbing.

Frank   6

I'm at work, talking to a child who's been referred for counseling. I share a room with another psychologist who's also interviewing a child. I'm taking notes while the child talks because I have to fill out long reports on each case. My legs hurt a lot and so do my hips.

Jack   5
I'm in my office. I'm having my second cup of coffee and lighting my fifth cigarette. I'm dictating a letter to my secretary. I'd call my pain medium: my legs are throbbing and my hands feel like electric current is passing through them.

Hannah   10
I'm in bed. I get up very early, and my daughter brings me breakfast at nine. Then I get back on the bed. Every morning a good friend of mine calls at nine-thirty. All that has already happened. The pain is un-believable; all I can do is sit up in bed. I'm reading a very good book.

Self-Portrait 3: How Are You?

It's still 10 A.M. Whether you're at work or at home, imagine that the phone rings or that someone walks up to you and says, "Hi, how are you?" Let this person be someone you know well but not intimately, a friend or co-worker who knows about your pain. After reading the other self-portraits describe your response in the space provided. Try to be as faithful as you can to how you would actually react.

Rosalie   "Fine, how are you?"
Everyone here knows about the accident, but I don't think it's right to talk about my personal problems at work. There are a lot of other things to my life besides

my pain, and I don't want people to relate to me just in terms of the accident.

Paul   **"Fine."**
I usually say *fine* because I know it impresses people that I'm so together when they know what I'm going through.

Edna   **"Awful."**
I guess there's no point hiding it, so I just come out and say it. Everyone who calls me knows how bad my pain is.

Frank   **"Oh, not bad. Could be worse."**
People know I'm in pain because of my short leg; they can see how hard it is for me to walk. I don't try to hide it, so I say how I'm feeling. I'd rather be asked how I am because that way I don't sound like I'm complaining.

Jack   **"Lousy, how are you?"**
I'm pretty straightforward about my pain, but I don't like to talk about it. If I say *lousy* right off the bat then he doesn't ask about my health. We get right down to business.

Hannah   **"I'm bearing it, but I've stopped grinning. How are you?"**
What do you expect? Everybody knows I have arthritis. How can you hide it when you can't walk? I try to make light of it and then we go on to talk about more important things.

▶ "_____"

Self-Portrait 4: The Attitudes Behind the Actions

Almost everyone with chronic pain has developed a philosophy for coping, an attitude that explains why he or she reacts to pain a certain way. Read the six other portraits first, then describe your own attitude toward pain as clearly and succinctly as you can.

Rosalie
I'm from pioneer stock, and I guess to me pain is a challenge just like any other. You have to make the best of it. I also believe that things happen to you for a reason. I see my pain as showing me the truth, so I accept it for what it can teach me. I'm pretty optimistic, in that I don't believe it will last longer than it has to.

Paul
I don't have a set philosophy. I try to fight it up to a point because I don't think you gain anything from giving in. But I like to vary the macho role with a little bit of sad sack every once in a while, otherwise I never get any sympathy.

Edna
I try to be brave but it's so hard. I believe pain is a punishment for your sins. You have to take it because the Lord sent it. I feel guilty because I'm not able to bear it as a good Christian ought to. Being able to take pain is a sign of goodness within.

Frank
My attitude is it's just one more part of life — not a very pleasant part, but that's the way it is. You take the bad with the good. There's no point trying to fight it. There's a certain virtue to taking things in stride.

Jack
I take an antagonist view of pain. To me it's like a war game. I will fight this goddamn thing till... till whatever. That's my whole approach, pure and simple. I try to neutralize it in my mind, never refer to pain as he — always an it. Pain is the enemy.

Hannah
I try to fight it. To me it's a question of dignity. I don't want to be pitied, so I don't want anyone to be able to see my suffering. I try as hard as I can to cover it up, and when I can't I don't let anyone come see me.

Seeing from the Eye of the Storm

Many people implicitly compare pain to a storm: "I guess I'll just have to ride it out"; "I'll weather it somehow." Each new bout can seem to strike with the sudden thrust of a tornado. When pain persists over days or weeks, it rattles and batters and shatters our innermost selves as violently as any tempest. Yet in the midst of our swirling emotions and physical pain, in the eye of the storm, there is calm. This is where I would like you to imagine yourself right now as you turn to Self-Portrait 5. The eye of the storm is an eye we all have, a far-seeing inner eye that sees with equanimity and depth no matter how chaotically life swirls around it. As you learn to see with the eye of the storm you will feel as if you have added a high-powered lens to your everyday vision.

Self-Portrait 5: The Feelings Below the Surface

Everybody, no matter how successful he or she may seem to be at handling pain, has a complex *emotional* reaction to being in pain and to the life changes pain so often brings with it. Because we have been taught to keep these personal, intimate, even embarrassing feelings private, we often aren't even aware of their existence. (When you're operating on "automatic cope" you can sometimes get by for years, as Jack did with the tough-man strategy borrowed from his wartime combat experience.) Pushing your feelings under doesn't make them go away; in fact, as you probably know from personal experience, sooner or later they start demanding attention.

As you read the six self-portraits below, return in your mind to where you usually are at 10 A.M. on a weekday morning. What are you feeling deep inside as you go about whatever you are doing? What is your *emotional* response? In the space provided, begin your self-portrait with the key mood word that best describes your overall feeling. Then develop your response by explaining why you think you feel that way. Let *recognition* be your guide.

Rosalie

I'm worried. After the accident I was very shaken up. In a way I accepted it; I thought maybe I needed that kind of close call. I still believe that, but I didn't expect the pain to last this long. I haven't been getting any better after all the physical therapy, and I'm starting to wonder if I ever will. I feel I've paid my dues

---

for that relationship. But now that I'm ready to move on, I can't go out and meet people like a normal woman my age.

Paul

I'm angry and worried. This is a hell of a thing to happen to a guy in the prime of life. I didn't think I overstressed my back, but apparently I did. Having a bad back makes me feel like a real failure. I used to be able to do just about anything. I was on top of the world. Now I feel like an old man. I'm still managing to make a living, but I'm up to my neck in debts from the six months I was out of work. The way my back has been feeling recently, I'm worried that it's going to cave in on me again.

Edna

I'm depressed. The pain has ruined my life. I can't work anymore and I feel completely worthless. Because of me my whole family is in debt. I'm ashamed to show my face in church because I know people are thinking things about me. I don't blame them. I know I have to pull myself together, but I can't. I feel like I brought this on myself, even though I didn't do it deliberately. I'm afraid my husband will leave me, and I wouldn't blame him if he did.

Frank

I guess I'm pretty much resigned after all these years. I know the pain isn't going to go away. But the pain in my hands has been getting much worse. I really don't see how I can keep working, since my job involves so much writing. But I can't afford to retire early. I have three kids to see through college. All that has me pretty worried. If I feel this bad at fifty-two, what's going to happen as I get older?

Jack
I'm frightened. Maybe it's age or something. I just don't think I can keep this up much longer. I'm not the kind of guy to take the easy way out, but the other day I finally asked my doctor for some codeine. With this thing moving into my hands now it's really getting to me. I have to get to work an hour early now just to keep up with the work load. If you want to know the truth, I'm scared out of my mind. I wonder what's going to become of me. Maybe it's not gout; maybe it's cancer.

Hannah
I'm angry. Over and over I ask myself why this should have to happen. I don't ask for a lot, but at my age it seems unbelievable that I should have to suffer so much. I know I'm very lucky to have such a wonderful family, but the shock of so much pain day after day is very hard to take. I'm very upset that I can't go to concerts anymore and that I have to be so dependent on my daughter.

Glancing back over these last self-portraits, you can probably identify a dominant response for each of them, including your own. Fear would have to head the list, followed by worry, especially about money and job security.

Guilt is harder for people to express, but if you look closely, you can see that it plays an important part in the emotional responses of Rosalie, Hannah, Edna, and Paul. Self-pity, even more difficult to speak about because it is so unacceptable in our society, is reflected in almost all the first six self-portraits, particularly in the last lines. Which emotions are most significant in your own Self-Portrait? Were you aware of them before?

The Pain Compounders

Warning: The following emotions can be dangerous to your health: self-pity, guilt, shame, embarrassment, worry, fear, anxiety, depression. If it's 10 A.M. on a typical weekday and your pain is in full swing *and* you're feeling any of these emotions, you're in trouble. You're also in good company. Along with Rosalie, Paul, Jack, and the others, you're a typical person in chronic pain. There's plenty you can do to reduce your pain once you recognize these common responses to pain for what they are: pain compounders.

What Are Pain Compounders?

A pain compounder is an emotion that has the same effect on pain as the weight of a human foot on the gas pedal of a car. Let's say your pain level is a 2 on the Plain Ordinary Pain Scale (see page 34). Add any one of the pain compounders and you can sit back and watch your pain soar to a solid 6 or 7.

Why are self-pity, guilt, shame, embarrassment, worry, fear, anxiety, and depression all pain compounders? Because all eight are immobilizing. They turn your energy inward rather than outward, which means that their full impact comes down on you, and down on your pain. The pain compounders are "down" emotions. Pity, guilt, shame, and embarrassment are forms of self-hatred. Worry, anxiety, and fear are energetic reactions that have no outlet: steam in your kettle. Depression can be the result of any or all of the other pain compounders.

The following mnemonic device may help you keep them in mind:

Pain Grows So Easily When Feelings Are Down.

(Self-Pity, Guilt, Shame, Embarrassment, Worry, Fear, Anxiety, Depression)

How Do Pain Compounders Work?

Numerous studies have revealed a definite link between fear and anxiety and increased sensitivity to pain. Apparently these emotions are powerful enough to trigger the fight-or-flight response. When you are afraid or anxious about your pain, for whatever reason, your body instinctively moves into a state of alert: your heart pumps faster, your adrenaline output increases, and your muscles tighten in readiness for flight or combat. But if you're sitting at a desk or your kitchen table or lying in bed, you aren't fighting or fleeing. You're mobilized for a defense that isn't going to take place. What you get is a lot of unnecessary, pain-provoking bodily tension that you can ill afford, creating more fear, anxiety, and all the other pain compounders. By identifying these responses individually and realizing that they are not a part of pain but something you bring *to* pain, you will begin to acquire a concrete sense of the key issues you need to address on your personal path to pain control.

The Question Mark of Pain

One reason the pain compounders play such a major role in most people's reactions to pain is because pain raises so many questions, from the nitty-gritty, practical ones such as how to cash your paycheck if you can't stand on line in the bank to the more far-reaching ones such as how to make a living if your back doesn't get better, or how you can raise two kids alone while suffering from rheumatoid arthritis. In his book *Medical Nemesis* Ivan Illich calls pain "the sign for something not answered." What is really wrong? Isn't there anything else that might work? These are the intrinsic questions pain continuously asks. The specific responses that compound *your* pain are really questions in disguise.

Most of us have learned a shortcut for getting from one end of life to the other: we tune out rather than in, leaving our questions, along with our participles, dangling. Fortunately, that doesn't work with chronic pain. I say *fortunately*, because if there's one thing chronic pain can teach us it's that there are no shortcuts: not in life, and not in pain. In my experience, if we don't train ourselves to answer the questions in the back of our minds *as they arise*, they begin to pile up. There they have nothing to do but molder. When questions pile up, they transmogrify into fear, guilt, worry, and all the other pain compounders. Nagging fears, gnawing doubts — these are feelings that eat away at you and undermine your strength, feelings that increase your pain while they decrease your ability to do anything about it. Pain compounders can't compound when *recognition* becomes an ongoing skill in your pain repertoire. By answering the questions behind your pain as quickly as you can, you keep your best energy free — for life.

Here are some of the specific questions you might ask based on the five self-portraits you have just completed:

- What's wrong with me? Do I fully understand the cause of my pain? If so, have I fully explored all the available treatments and made an informed choice? Have I found something that helps, at least to some extent?

- Do I take all the steps I could to reduce my pain? Am I involved in activities that make it worse?

- Is my attitude toward pain helping or hindering me?

- How do I come across to others in Self-Portrait 3? Is there a large gap between the way I behave when other people are around and the feelings that emerge in Self-Portrait 5? If so, what outlets do I have for expressing the feelings I keep below the surface?

- What are the main factors compounding my pain? What are my worst fears? Have I done everything I could to work them through? If not, what steps could I take?

These questions point the way to your path to pain control. You will want to keep them in mind as you turn to Chapter 4 to begin taking your pain apart so you can put yourself back together.

4

Taking Your Pain Apart
So You Can Put
Yourself Back Together

In Chapter 3 you learned to become an observer on your
own behalf, venturing into the "field" and returning again
and again to refine your impressions. You began to claim the
place called pain for yourself, clearing away unnecessary
preconceptions and recognizing the specific pain compounders that feed into your experience of pain. With recognition
as your guide, you were able to raise key questions that
point the way to your personal path to pain control.

Your experience of chronic pain, as we've already seen, is
the result of a very complicated and intriguing relationship:
the interaction between a given medical condition (yours)
and a given personality (yours). Because the mind-body interaction is constantly changing, both your physical condition and your emotional response not only to pain but to
everything else go through many phases over time, even
varying from hour to hour. All these subtle shifts have a

profound impact on the experience of chronic pain. The more you know about both sides of the mind-body equation, the more effectively you'll be able to chart your personal path to pain control. By learning to identify the different forces that converge in your pain, you can learn to change the balance. When you change the balance you change your pain. You can make it worse, or you can reduce it. Once you have the choice, you are in control.

The first stage of coping is pain reduction. To this end, we're going to focus now on the two sides of the pain equation for an in-depth analysis of the way mind and body interact in your pain. In this chapter we'll look at your present medical situation with a set of charts designed to show you exactly where you can make simple adjustments in your daily routine that can significantly reduce your pain. In Chapter 5 we'll turn our attention to the major social and cultural factors that directly affect your experience of pain, also with a view toward recognizing specific areas that can be modified.

By taking your pain apart, you're dividing what is of course an indivisible whole — the mind-body relationship. There is a logical reason for this. As you deconstruct your pain, you will simultaneously be reconstructing your attitudes and expectations. The process is simple, but the effect is extraordinary. When you have looked at both halves of your pain equation in detail, the pain you put back together will be very different from the one you took apart. Most important of all, you will be different, because you will have learned to make the complicity of mind and body work *for* you instead of against you. Many of the questions you raised at the end of Chapter 3 will have been effortlessly answered, and you'll be in a much better position to answer those that remain.

In this chapter, without leaving *recognition* behind, we expand your expertise by adding *responsibility,* the second of the three R's of pain control, to your coping repertoire. As you will come to understand in the following pages, taking responsibility for your pain is a giant step on the path to pain control.

What Is Responsibility?

The word *responsibility* is most often used in a moralistic sense, especially in describing negative events: the man *responsible* for the crime, for example. You are not responsible for your pain in this sense of the word. You didn't cause it, and you have no reason to feel guilty for it. This may be hard to accept, because the association between pain and punishment is deeply embedded in our culture. Even our word *pain* comes from the Latin *poena,* meaning "punishment." "Pain and being guilty, being hurt — it all goes together," one woman told me. Although she had been injured in a car driven by someone else, *she* felt guilty. Another woman, an inveterate jogger whose aching shinbone fractured as she crossed a finish line and then failed to knit, felt that she was being punished for her willfulness. "I should have stopped," she told me. "One of the nightmares I have to live with is that I did this to myself. I didn't listen to my body."

Recently, the idea of pain as punishment has been given a modern twist in a number of books and articles that claim a direct connection between personality and illness. You get what you are, according to this latter-day doomsday theory of disease. If you read even a few of the articles on the "cancer-prone personality," the "M.S. personality," or the "rheumatoid arthritis personality," you may wonder, as I did, why all the patients sound the same. In *Illness as Metaphor* Susan Sontag questioned the basic science behind the idea of a link between personality and illness:

Scarcely a week passes without a new article announcing to some general public or other the scientific link between cancer and painful feelings. Investigations are cited — most articles refer to the same ones — in which, out of, say, several hundred cancer patients, two-thirds or three-fifths report being depressed or unsatisfied with their lives, and having suffered from the loss (through death or rejection or separation) of a parent, lover, spouse, or close friend. But it seems likely that out of several hundred people who do *not* have cancer, most would also report depressing emotions and past traumas: this is called the human condition.

The psychologists of illness have taken the mind-body connection to its illogical extreme. If you were to believe their studies, any change in your life, whether good or bad (including death, marriage, divorce, college graduation, moving), puts your health in jeopardy. The more changes in a given year, the more stress and the higher your risk of illness. A British social scientist, Richard Totman, has even gone so far as to propose that illness is a kind of biological punishment — nature's revenge — that is visited upon those members of society who deviate from an evolutionary norm. That norm, he suggests in all seriousness, is mediocrity; mutations (those who move, marry, divorce, change jobs) fall sick or hurt themselves in order to keep the rest of the species on its proper track.

Such short-circuit thinking blithely ignores the existence of germs and viruses, not to mention the perils of modern transportation, the hazards of the industrial work place, and the fearsome pollution of nearly every segment of our environment. The air we breathe, the water we drink, and the meals we put on our tables — and thus our very cells — have all been contaminated through toxic chemicals, radioactive nuclear waste, and the preservatives that are pumped into our food. These recent additions to the ecosystem, along with the materials in which we clothe ourselves and out of which we build and equip our schools, homes, offices, and hospitals, will surely have worse long-term consequences for human health than any ills we have seen to date. We would do far better as a society to examine the links between cancer and toxic chemicals, or between food additives and lowered resistance to disease, than between illness and personality. Yet people still take comfort in looking inward for the explanations of their own poor health. Why?

According to Dr. Eric J. Cassell, author of *The Healer's Art,* psychological explanations of illness allow patients "to fix the blame on the most comforting locus of all — themselves. Why this is the most advantageous source of blame lies at the heart of a feature of illness that is most disturbing to the sick person: the loss of control. If the person is the source of his illness he remains in control, even if it is a perverse kind of control." Perverse it is, because self-blame creates perverse illusions. If you tied the knot, you can untie it. By analogy, if your personality caused your arthritis, then with a little overhaul — or a few years on the couch — you should be as good as new. Illness just isn't that simple. Some events *are* out of our control (a car coming at you from the other side of a highway, a virus that sweeps a whole town). Most of the time chance is as much to blame as necessity in bringing about an injury or illness. However, while you may not be responsible for causing your pain, you *can* choose to be responsible for reducing it. That way, to use an old cliché, you won't be adding insult to injury.

Responsibility in this sense of the word means "the ability to respond": responsiveness. When it comes to chronic pain, responsibility can exist only in the presence of knowledge, because you are able to respond most fully only when you are informed and aware. No matter how much others want to help you, and no matter how much you might wish them to, no one else on earth can or will respond to your pain, because no one else can ever know it as you do, from the inside. By committing yourself to being responsible for your pain, you commit yourself to learning everything you can about it and following through on your knowledge with action.

Owning Your Pain from A to Z

As a person with chronic pain, you want to know everything you possibly can about your medical situation. Medical ignorance is one of pain's chief enemies, perhaps the greatest pain compounder of them all. It increases your anxiety, your fear, your dependence on doctors, and your ability to plan your life in a coherent way, which in turn can dramatically affect your relationships with friends and loved ones and even jeopardize your income. Any one of these consequences of medical ignorance can actually increase your pain. When, in Dr. Cassell's words, "lack of understanding threatens our completeness and exposes us to unknown dangers, we make new and repeated interpretations with added emotional content to compensate for a deficient reality." As we saw in Chapters 2 and 3, added emotional content can translate into added pain. One more time: however you chose to manage your life before you were in pain, you can't afford to carry any extra weight around now. Loose ends and nagging questions must be taken care of as they appear, or they will wreak havoc on your pain.

The Importance of a Diagnosis
Part of taking responsibility for your pain is making sure that you've done everything feasible to obtain an accurate diagnosis of your condition. You may have to figure out a few things about yourself before you tackle this one. There are some people who would truly rather not know what is wrong with them. If you are such a person, you may feel

that if you knew what you had (assuming your condition is as terrible as you think it is), you would be even worse off. Think hard about your choice of ignorance. Your fear of the truth may be holding you back from taking a few simple, important steps that could make a big difference in how you feel.

Contrary to popular opinion, a diagnosis won't let you see into a crystal ball and know exactly what is going to happen to you over time as the result of a particular illness or injury. Nor will it be a ticket to a cure. All a diagnosis tells you is what you have, based on how closely your condition resembles an ideal disease construct that physicians have established through research, observation, and treatment.

If, for example, you have rheumatoid arthritis, you are one of 6.5 million people in the United States with that disease. Each one of those 6.5 million cases is unique; each has its individual characteristics derived from both the person's biochemical makeup (itself a complex product of heredity and environment) and his or her whole past and present experience. A doctor cannot say — or shouldn't — "You have RA, therefore ... X." What a practiced physician can do, however, is listen to each patient and help create a responsible approach to managing the illness.

Why is it so important to have a diagnosis if it doesn't tell you what's going to become of you? First of all, because it tells you what you *don't* have. Once you are able to lay your doubts and fears to rest, you will have removed one of the major obstacles — and pain compounders — from your path to pain control. Secondly, a diagnosis can point the way to specific modes of treatment.

It May Not Be Easy
If you don't know what's wrong with you and no one else seems to be able to figure it out, you're in for a tough

time. Where ignorance exists, fear persists. Every dire illness you've ever heard of or managed to read about runs
wild through your imagination, over and over, around and
around, invading your peace of mind and compounding your
pain.

In addition, once a thorough medical workup has been
obtained from a reasonably prestigious hospital and still no
diagnosis results, you become a prime target for an accusation the medical establishment is apt to make when it fails
to diagnose. You become "crazy" until proven sick. (This,
by the way, is far more likely to happen if you are a woman,
as we'll see in Chapter 5.) Such a reputation can make it
very hard for you to get serious medical attention. I know
what that's like, because it happened to me. It was close to
three years before I found a doctor who was able to pinpoint the cause of my pain and devise an effective approach
for managing my illness. In the meantime I was warned repeatedly by friends, family, and even other physicians that
if I accumulated too thick a record I would soon be looked
upon as an undesirable patient whenever I set foot in a
prospective doctor's office. This I found to be shamefully
true. It's a real Catch-22. When you're undiagnosed for more
than six months, your search for a diagnosis begins to be
held against you.

Still, no matter what people tell you, you have to be cou-
rageous. If *you* are convinced that there is something physically wrong with you, keep going until you find a doctor
who can help you. Your perseverance will eventually be
rewarded.

Some words of advice: read Chapter 10, "Dealing with
Doctors," before you make your next appointment with a
new physician. If you need encouragement, read some of
the books marked with an asterisk on the Suggested Reading List beginning on page 243.

Your Pain Profile

Whenever you go to a new doctor you're asked, "Well, what seems to be the trouble?" Your medical history can sound to you like a broken record after a while. But have you ever given *yourself* your medical history? The questionnaire on pages 58–59 will provide you with a detailed medical chart for your own information and future reference. Where you don't know or don't remember something, check the appropriate box — and take note. The chart will clarify key aspects of your physical condition, including those areas requiring further research or observation.

Putting the Final Touches on Your Pain Profile

Now that you've filled out Your Medical History and laid out the broad lines of your pain, it's time to give your medical profile a little nuance. Most people's pain isn't always exactly the same day in and day out, minute after agonizing minute. Quite often there are subtle variations even within a given hour. When their pain lessens or intensifies, many people can trace these changes — at least to some degree — to a whole range of quite specific factors. Can you? By learning to identify them one by one, you may be able to intervene quite specifically to diminish your pain, because all these areas, except the weather, are eminently suited to control.

Some of the key influences on pain, depending on your underlying condition, are time of day, regularity of sleep, amount and quality of sleep, atmospheric temperature, humidity or dryness, barometric pressure, altitude, transportation, rest, exercise, and direct application of heat or cold via wet packs, ice packs, heating pads, saunas, baths, whirlpools, or swimming. Nutrition can play a large part too,

Your Medical History

Today's Date _____

Your Pain Level Right Now (see page 34) _____

Diagnosis _____

Site(s) of pain _____

Approximate date of onset _____ Age at onset _____

How long have you had chronic pain? _____

Is your pain ☐ constant? ☐ episodic? ☐ infrequent?
☐ other? (specify) _____

Is your pain the result of an accident or injury?
☐ Yes; ☐ No; ☐ Don't know; ☐ Maybe.
If yes, give details:

Is your pain the result of a hereditary condition?
☐ Yes; ☐ No; ☐ Don't know; ☐ Maybe.
If yes, are other members of your family affected?
Enumerate:

Have you experienced any periods of remission since the
onset of your present condition?

_____ Number of major remissions   Dates and duration

From: _____   To: _____
From: _____   To: _____
From: _____   To: _____
From: _____   To: _____
From: _____   To: _____

Which of the following best describes your pain? Check
all applicable terms:

☐ Burning	☐ Crushing	☐ Stabbing
☐ Throbbing	☐ Boring	☐ Searing
☐ Grinding	☐ Gnawing	☐ Wrenching

☐ Shooting	☐ Blinding	☐ Aching
☐ Pounding	☐ Tearing	☐ Drawing

What, if any, medication(s) are you currently taking for relief of pain and pain-associated symptoms (stiffness, muscle spasms, inflammation, etc.)? List all drugs, both prescription and over-the-counter.

Name of Drug	Daily Dosage	Complete	Significant	Partial	Minimal	None
1. _____	___	___	___	___	___	___
2. _____	___	___	___	___	___	___
3. _____	___	___	___	___	___	___
4. _____	___	___	___	___	___	___
5. _____	___	___	___	___	___	___
6. _____	___	___	___	___	___	___
7. _____	___	___	___	___	___	___
8. _____	___	___	___	___	___	___
9. _____	___	___	___	___	___	___
10. _____	___	___	___	___	___	___

The "Degree of Relief" columns above are headed: Complete, Significant, Partial, Minimal, None.

What other treatments, if any, have you explored for relief of pain and associated symptoms? Check those you have already tried, indicating degree of relief obtained.

	Complete	Significant	Partial	Minimal	None
☐ Acupuncture	___	___	___	___	___
☐ Biofeedback	___	___	___	___	___
☐ Chiropractic	___	___	___	___	___
☐ Herbal Medicine	___	___	___	___	___
☐ Homeopathy	___	___	___	___	___
☐ Hypnosis	___	___	___	___	___
☐ Massage	___	___	___	___	___
☐ Meditation	___	___	___	___	___
☐ Nutrition	___	___	___	___	___
☐ Transcutaneous Nerve Stimulation	___	___	___	___	___

particularly the intake of coffee, alcohol, nicotine, marijuana, other mind-altering drugs, food additives, and, in some cases, salt and sugar.

Try to be as precise as you can as you fill out the Pain Inventory on page 61. The more accurately you spell out these "external" influences on your pain, the more intelligently you'll be able to pinpoint feasible changes.

Taking Responsibility: The Follow-Up

Responsibility doesn't stop at the point where knowledge trails off into ignorance. That's where it begins. The next step is following through on your Pain Inventory with the simple changes that will begin to shift the balance between mind and body, easing up on your pain and thereby taking some of the burden (pain compounders) off your mind.

Let's say you've figured out that your pain is more severe in the morning when you first get up and that heat provides a fair amount of relief. You have to be out of the house at seven o'clock every morning because your job begins at eight, an hour away from where you live. Why not alter your morning routine to accommodate your stiffness and take advantage of your pain's responsiveness to soothing heat? You might need to get up half an hour earlier to make time for a slow bath (perhaps accompanied by your favorite relaxation exercise* or some gentle music), so you'll have to balance that adjustment against your sleep requirements. These are decisions that only you can make, based on the copious testimony you have just provided yourself.

Many people notice that their cigarette consumption doubles or even triples when they're in a lot of pain. "The worse the pain is, the more I smoke," was a recurring theme in

---

* The Pain Emergency Kit on pages 209–226 will give you some easy-to-learn ideas, if this is an area you haven't yet explored.

Your Pain Inventory   Today's Date _____

Generally speaking, when is your pain at its worst (W) and when at its best (B)? Immediately on Rising_____; Morning _____; Afternoon_____; Early Evening_____; Late Evening _____; No Particular Time_____; Don't Know_____.

How often does pain interfere with your sleep?
☐ Often; ☐ Rarely; ☐ Never.

How much sleep do you need on an average night? _____

If the time you get to sleep is important, at what time do you need to get to sleep? _____

If you get less than this amount, what is the effect on your pain? _____

Do you have trouble sleeping for reasons other than pain? If yes, specify: _____

How do the following affect your pain?	Makes It Worse	Improves It	No Change	Don't Know
Cold weather	____	____	____	____
Hot weather	____	____	____	____
Humidity	____	____	____	____
Dryness	____	____	____	____
Barometric pressure	____	____	____	____
Change of seasons	____	____	____	____
Altitude	____	____	____	____

Is your pain increased by any of these modes of travel? ☐ Car; ☐ Bus; ☐ Boat; ☐ Train; ☐ Plane. Do you know why?

How do the following affect your pain? Mark with a + those that help; use a − sign for those that have no effect or a negative one; NT for Not Tried. Hot bath or shower_____; Sauna_____; Heating pad_____; Cold bath or shower_____; Whirlpool_____; Ice pack_____; Other (Specify) _____

If your pain is alleviated by any of the following, mark with a + sign. If exercise is helpful, specify the type(s) you have tried:

☐ Rest; ☐ Elevation of Limbs; ☐ Exercise. _____

	Yes	No	Amount Daily	Decreases Pain	Increases Pain
Do you smoke cigarettes?	____	____	____	____	____
Do you drink?	____	____	____	____	____
Do you smoke marijuana or use any other mind-altering drugs? (Specify)	____	____	____	____	____

the interviews I did for this book. In addition to its notorious effects on the heart and lungs, nicotine constricts the blood vessels. If your pain is due to an inflammatory condition or a cardiovascular problem, you would be wise to give up cigarettes for good.*

Remember, there is no good or bad behavior when it comes to chronic pain. There is up-and-down behavior, actions, and attitudes that lift you out of pain, and those that pull you deeper into it. It is a question of *choosing*.

The simple chart below may help you to make sense of what you know and to devise a plan of action that will start you on your way toward pain control.

Do I have a diagnosis? ☐ Yes; ☐ No. If no, why not?

_____

If yes, have I tried the currently available treatments for my condition? ☐ Yes; ☐ No.

Three factors that definitely *increase* my pain:	Three factors that definitely *decrease* my pain:
1. _____	1. _____
2. _____	2. _____
3. _____	3. _____
Are these part of my daily routine? ☐ Yes; ☐ No.	Are these part of my daily routine? ☐ Yes; ☐ No.
Can they be *eliminated?* ☐ Yes; ☐ No.	Can they be *added?* ☐ Yes; ☐ No.

Let's assume for a moment, via a generous leap of the imagination, that your medical knowledge is now as complete as it can be and that you've learned habitually to take

* The U.S. Government Department of Health and Human Services publishes an excellent booklet called "Calling It Quits." It worked for me — I stopped in October 1979, and I'm still not smoking. For a free copy, write to the Public Health Service, National Institutes of Health, Bethesda, MD 20014.

every conceivable measure to reduce your pain based on the plan of action you've charted on page 62. You still have pain, but you've made some genuine progress and acted responsibly on your medical knowledge.

Personal, cultural, and socioeconomic factors are just as influential as physical ones in shaping your experience of pain. Such determinants as childhood illness, your sex, ethnic background, present job status, income, and age are a few of the ingredients we'll be discussing in Chapter 5 as we look at the other side of the mind-body equation.

▪ 5

Putting Your Pain in Context

> On the morning of the third day, the pain returned
> home bringing all of its kinfolk. Not that any single
> one of them was overwhelming, but just that all in
> concert, or even in small repertory groups, they were
> excruciating.
>
> AUDRE LORDE,
> *The Cancer Journals*

Pain does not exist in the abstract. It exists as part of a
medical condition, and it exists within a whole network of
factors that affect your reaction to it. People can and do
react to the "identical" amount of pain differently, depending on the situation they're in. For example, if a good friend
gives you a playful pat on the back, your reaction will be
quite different from what it would be if a total stranger hit
you from behind with the same force. The key word is *context*. In some cultures, extremely painful initiation rites are
endured without any sign of suffering, presumably because
the pain is seen to be serving a higher purpose.

But context can also increase pain, as it did for Tolstoy's
hero Ivan Ilyich, the bureaucrat whose death and dying

were never acknowledged by his family: "His ache, this dull gnawing ache that never ceased for a moment, seemed to have acquired a new and more serious significance from the doctor's remarks. Ivan Ilyich now watched it with a new and oppressive feeling." Ivan Ilyich was never told that he had cancer, but Tolstoy so masterfully evokes the atmosphere of secrecy and dread surrounding his illness that we, like Ilyich himself, know that he is dying.

The Vietnam veteran who returns disabled from a war that was profoundly questioned may bear his scars — and chronic pain — quite differently from the veteran of World War II who returned home to a hero's welcome.

What this all adds up to is that pain is relative. When it comes to pain and illness, we would all, doctors and patients alike, do well to remember Dr. William Osler's dictum that it's more important "to know what patient has a disease than what disease a patient has."

To complicate matters even further, pain does not exist in one context alone; it exists in many — as many contexts as there are aspects in your life. If it's true, as Shakespeare said, that all the world's a stage and that we are merely players, we're in a very complex play indeed. Not only are there billions of players whose roles can overlap, but each separate one of us is simultaneously acting in an incredible number of plays. It's like standing on many different stages at once, all on different levels. Some of the wonder and some of life's deepest experiences stem from the overlapping of these different plays we're in, these different contexts. But in pain, matters tend less to be wonderful and more to be terribly confused. In order to sort out our strengths and weaknesses and keep going on the path to pain control, we need to be aware of the major contexts in which pain, for want of a better phrase, takes place.

By examining the central, most important contexts one by one, you'll be able to see exactly how and where they overlap, where they conflict, and whether, on balance, your overall attitude toward pain is helping or hindering you. By applying the principles of recognition and responsibility to this side of the pain equation, you will be able, just as you did in Chapter 4, to pinpoint the specific small changes that will add up to major change and, ultimately, pain control.

Because we are social creatures, pain derives much of its complexity from the multi-tiered social reality in which we live. All of us are members of a family, whether or not that family remained intact over the years. We are also male or female, and, due to the legacy of divergent cultural conditioning for the two sexes, our gender has a strong impact on our response to pain and illness. In addition, we are members of a religious or ethnic group with specific cultural values that, whether we accept or reject them, play an important role in shaping our outlook on the world. Our financial situation, age, and current living arrangements also interact to affect our experience of pain. The degree to which each of these different contexts affects *your* pain is something only you can determine after you have carefully weighed each one in the balance of your judgment.

A Flash to the Past

What is your earliest memory of pain? How old were you and what caused the pain? Who stayed with you, or didn't? What was the underlying message — sympathy, punishment, annoyance, anger? How did you feel — comforted, rejected, guilty, afraid? Were you expected to be brave, encouraged to express your feelings, allowed to cry, treated tenderly or harshly? Unlocking such early recollections can provide important clues in understanding the way you respond to pain today. A study of attitudes toward dental care found that family experience and attitudes were the single most important factors affecting an adult's behavior in the dentist's chair. Take a look at your own past. If every scraped knee was the occasion for a kiss from your mother or a close relative, you may have a strong association between pain and attention, or pain and affection. (I say "may" because there are no hard and fast rules.) Pain takes us back to our earliest, most intimate experience of suffering.

When I interviewed Jack, he told me of a shocking experience he had had two weeks before. His gout had been acting up and, at one point, to his utter amazement, he heard his own voice cry out, "Ma, take it away!" His mother has been dead for twenty years. To Jack this experience was both disturbing and humiliating. But when we talked about it, he began to see why he had called out to his mother in a night of agony. Pain and illness make us feel helpless and dependent, taking us back in a flash to primal, often long-forgotten feelings.

Jack's association was between pain and his mother's tenderness. But for other people, a very different pattern can prevail. In some families pain and illness may be met with impatience, anger, or disapproval. This can be on moral grounds or may perhaps be just a question of temperament. It can also reflect economic hardship. One woman I interviewed, whom I'll call Frances, grew up in a large farm family in Utah in which "if you complained, you damned well better be good and sick" because a visit to the doctor meant financial strain. The children learned to keep their aches and pains to themselves and spoke up only when they needed serious medical attention. Frances and her siblings, all of whom have had major health problems stemming from the nuclear testing of the early 1950s, still battle with the sense of guilt that they associate with illness, even though they all know rationally that they are not to blame for their medical troubles.

Great writers often have a gift for conjuring up the world

of childhood in words that penetrate the very core of memory. This is how the German writer Rainer Maria Rilke described childhood illness in a passage of *The Notebooks of Malte Laurids Brigge,* his fictionalized autobiography:

> As I listened to the hot, flaccid stuttering on the other side of the partition, . . . for the first time in many, many years it was there again. That which had struck into me my first, profound terror, when as a child I lay ill with fever: The Big Thing. Yes, that was what I had always called it, when they stood around my bed and felt my pulse and asked me what had frightened me: The Big Thing. And when they got the doctor and he came and spoke to me, I begged him only to make The Big Thing go away . . . It was there like a huge, dead beast that had once, when it was still alive, been my hand or my arm.

Rilke's fearful memory of illness contrasts with the tender, reassuring scene described by the novelist Toni Morrison in *The Bluest Eye:*

> But was it really like that? As painful as I remember? Only mildly. Or rather, it was a productive and fructifying pain. Love, thick and dark as Alaga syrup, eased up into that cracked window. I could smell it — taste it — sweet, musty, with an edge of wintergreen in its base — everywhere in that house. It stuck, along with my tongue, to the frosted windowpanes. It coated my chest, along with the salve, and when the flannel came undone in my sleep, the clear, sharp curves of air outlined its presence on my throat. And in the night, when my coughing was dry and tough, feet padded into the room, hands repinned the flannel, readjusted the quilt, and rested a moment on my forehead. So when I think of autumn, I think of somebody with hands who does not want me to die.

Our training in matters of survival begins so early — virtually from the moment of birth — that it would be impossible to retrace the steps of all those who watched over us, constantly on the alert to make sure we didn't fall, handle sharp objects, burn ourselves. If your memory is good enough, or if you've raised children yourself, you can probably think of dozens of small phrases ("Watch out, don't cut yourself"; "Look both ways before crossing"; "Careful — that's hot") that help to mold a child's consciousness of pain. But more than just warnings go into our pain-training years. We acquire attitudes and expectations, and we acquire a pain *style*.

Your pain style has to do with how you express your pain — whether you clam up and isolate yourself from those around you, as Jack does; whether you seek company, as Rosalie does; whether you moan and whimper, like Edna, or cover your anguish with a hearty laugh, like Hannah. Traits such as these often follow a family pattern. Was your family vocal and dramatic about pain, or was such behavior frowned upon? Do you yourself tend to be dramatic, or are you low-key in your expression of pain?

If your present pain-producing condition began in childhood, it may have affected your whole self-image. A man I'll call Arthur suffered serious heart damage at the age of seven as a result of rheumatic fever. Now forty-two, he has always done everything possible to keep his severe chest pain invisible to others. He carried with him into adult life his fear of being labeled "sick" and therefore excluded by "the other kids."

If an older or younger sibling or a parent or other adult member of your household was in chronic pain as you were growing up, that too may have affected your attitude toward your own pain. You may have admired the way the person dealt with pain. On the other hand, if you're remembering someone whose behavior was manipulative or arbitrary or frightening, you will have an entirely different set of associations. The possibilities are endless. The point is to recognize your reality and its roots in your family. Whether you follow or reject the "illness behavior" that was set before you, it was and is an important determinant of your own response to pain.

Gender

Closely related to early experience of pain and family attitudes toward illness is the striking difference in the pain behavior taught to, and expected of, boys and girls. This difference is deeply rooted and plays a major, often overlooked role in the way we experience our pain.

The Bible tells us that when God made Eve as a companion for Adam, he "caused a deep sleep to fall upon Adam" before removing the legendary rib. Nowhere in the Bible is there mention of any similar anesthesia for women. In fact, when anesthesia for the pains of childbirth was first introduced in the nineteenth century, its use was virulently opposed by both the Roman Catholic and Episcopal churches on the grounds that "woman's lot is to suffer." To this day many women readily see their pain, whether from childbirth, menstruation ("the curse"), or any other cause, as somehow their natural fate in life. According to an old adage, "Man endures pain as an undeserved punishment; woman accepts it as a natural heritage."

Generally speaking, in most Western countries males are taught to model themselves on soldiers, to be brave and "bite the bullet." We've all seen the screen-size Hollywood cowboy who barely flinches as the frontier doctor's rusty knife deftly frees the bullet lodged in his chest, only to rise with a terse "Thanks, Doc." "Boys don't cry" is the refrain that echoes on playgrounds around the world as little boys fall, get hurt, pick themselves up, and shake themselves off.

Little girls do cry, and they get hugged, kissed, and coddled for it. Expectations for emotional pain follow much the same pattern, with boys refining the art of stoicism during the very same years that girls are acquiring the art of "feeling deeply." Before they ever set foot in a classroom, boys and girls have learned two very different lessons about pain.

When some of these boys and girls grow up into men and women with chronic pain, their response to pain often mimics the sex-stereotyped behavior they learned as children. By proving how "strong" you are and how much pain you can "take," you're only asking for more. The same is true if you accept pain as your "lot" in life. These two attitudes are, respectively, the so-called masculine and feminine responses to pain that we've been taught since childhood.

On the basis of the handful of studies conducted so far, there is no scientific evidence to support the popular belief that women can stand more pain than men. There *is* evidence, however, that men's and women's divergent *attitudes* toward pain have a powerful influence not only on how individuals of both sexes express and experience their pain, but also on how their pain is viewed by others, including, often to their peril, the health professionals to whom they go for help.

In a 1971 experiment, when physicians were asked to describe the typical complaining patient, 72 percent of those responding spontaneously used "she." Only 4 percent used a male pronoun, while the remaining 24 percent gave a genderless description. Gena Corea, who reports this study in her ground-breaking book *The Hidden Malpractice*, concludes, "Men describe symptoms, it seems, but women 'complain.' "

A 1979 study published in the *Journal of the American Medical Association* asked male physicians to evaluate an equal number of male and female patients (fifty-two married couples). Researchers from the University of California at

San Diego, where the study was conducted, found that the doctors invariably ordered more extensive workups for the male patients than for female patients with the same complaints (back pain, headache, chest pain, dizziness, and fatigue).

A 1980 analysis of intake interviews at the Lourdes Hospital Pain Unit in Binghamton, New York, conducted by unit director Dr. Dorothea Lack, showed that prior to admission, female patients at the center had received more minor tranquilizers (mainly Valium and Librium) than male patients had. The same study also found that men entering the clinic had received twice as much pain-related surgery (nerve blocks, laminectomies, implantation of dorsal column stimulators) as women. While the value of these procedures might be questionable in many cases, Dr. Lack concluded that men's pain problems were more directly, specifically, and swiftly addressed than women's. (The smallest percentage of pain-related surgery in the Lourdes study was reported by housewives, who also averaged the longest duration of pain, at an average of 10.86 years, compared to 10.29 years for the total female sample and 7.46 years for the men.)

Results of a study of pain patients at Upstate Medical Center in Syracuse, New York, reported by Dr. Richard Phillips, associate professor of psychiatry at the center, showed that the women's average hospital stay was three days longer than the men's.

A survey of former outpatients of the West Virginia University Medical Center Pain Clinic in Morgantown, reported by Dr. Robert Pawlicki, associate director of the clinic, showed that women with chronic pain were significantly more likely than men to spend the whole day in bed and twice as likely as men to attribute their pain to "no known cause" (which means they either didn't understand their medical condition or hadn't been diagnosed).

Both the Morgantown and the Binghamton studies found men more likely than women to be receiving some form of financial assistance for their pain-related medical problem, whether in the form of workmen's compensation, Social Security disability payments, or welfare.

Putting all these findings together, a clear pattern emerges:

- Men's pain is more likely than women's to be taken more seriously sooner and to receive relatively early validation in the form of economic compensation.

- Women's pain is more likely than men's to be treated as if it were largely psychological (hence the preponderance of tranquilizers), and women are less likely than men to receive economic assistance while they are ill or disabled.

Women are at greater risk than men of being subjected to lingering hospital stays and debilitating treatment. It is easy to see that such a starkly differential situation can create and prolong an overload of such pain compounders as fear, anxiety, and depression for women who are not receiving adequate, specific care, who are not given clear explanations of their medical problems, and whose health-related financial difficulties go unrelieved.

Women who begin to crack under this trio of pressures are offered the helping hand of tranquilizers and sedatives, drawing them further into a cycle of depression and dependency from which escape becomes increasingly difficult.*

Doctors, apparently all too readily, assume that if a woman

---

* A few statistics from the 1978 hearings of the House Select Committee on Narcotics Abuse and Control show that 32 million American women compared to 19 million men have used tranquilizers prescribed by a doctor, and 16 million women as compared to 12 million men have used physician-prescribed sedatives. In 1977, 8.5 million women used tranquilizers and 3 million women used sedatives.

is sick it is because she is "frazzled," that if a woman is sick someone will take care of her, and that women are not a valuable part of the work force. These are crushing assumptions for a woman in pain to confront, especially since an estimated 18 percent of American households are currently headed by women, which means that a woman with disabling pain is often the sole source of support not only for herself but also for dependent children.

But the risks of mistreatment are by no means limited to women. Because men, to a greater degree than women, have learned to equate their sense of personal self-worth with their dollar value on the market, they have a double incentive, financial and personal, to return to work as soon as possible. This may, in part, account for the tens of thousands of major surgical procedures (laminectomies, spinal fusions) performed each year on men who, were society both more generous and less demanding, might benefit more (and wind up in much better shape) from more conservative treatment.

On the other hand, men are often viewed by doctors as suffering from an "overvalidation" of their pain. When their invalid status is confirmed through workmen's compensation or Social Security payments, some men are said to lose confidence in their ability to function productively and to become dependent and depressed as a result. The problem, of course, is not the economic compensation, which should be guaranteed to every person with chronic pain until he or she is able to resume productive work, but the fact that reentry into the job market is made so difficult for a person with medical problems. Our society keeps hundreds of thousands of people underutilized by ignoring their potential in new and untried skills. If disability payments were automatically accompanied by rehabilitation and retraining, as they are in New Zealand, where disabled workers can return to part-time jobs without forfeiting their entire compensation check (which is adjusted to reflect their earnings), doctors would have no excuse for looking down on men who get trapped in the compensation net.

Men have an additional problem when it comes to chronic pain. Some men, because the cultural message of male strength and invulnerability is so strong, have a tough time adjusting to whatever changes and limitations pain imposes on their lives. They may actually make their pain worse by fighting it, because as boys they were taught to fight and resist. In addition, since masculinity and physical prowess are so closely linked in our culture, they may even feel a loss of virility as a result of being in pain. A number of the men I interviewed expressed this feeling and were in great distress because of it. Impotence is not at all uncommon in men with chronic pain. Just as women have to learn to separate their female conditioning from their own experience of pain (it's one more inherited interpretation), it is essential for men to separate their male conditioning from their experience of pain. Even if there are certain kinds of work you can no longer do, that fact in no way reflects upon you as a man or, most importantly, as a human being.

Disabled Ironworker Awarded $2.2 Million

A 46-year-old disabled ironworker who became depressed and who "considered himself a failure" because he couldn't "bring home the bacon" was awarded $2.2 million by a Manhattan jury, his lawyer said.

The ironworker, Anthony T. of Staten Island, developed a "severe reactive depression" after he was hurt in a 12-foot fall while working on the 40th level of the Citicorp building in Manhattan on May 10, 197—, according to his lawyer.

The six-woman jury, in making the award in State Supreme Court, found that the general contractor and two subcontractors were negligent in the placement of a brace over which Mr. T. tripped just before he fell.

The recent news item above reflects all the gender issues that have just been discussed. In a different cultural context, Anthony T. might not have felt so worthless because of his disability; he might have been retrained, and his self-esteem would have returned. Now, with a $2.2 million dollar investment in depression and failure, what chance does he have of retrieving his ability to lead a productive life? Finally, would a full-time homemaker injured in a fall in her own home (where the vast majority of disabling injuries occur, according to the U.S. Department of Labor), ever receive financial compensation for her depression at no longer being able to "cook the bacon"?

Making a Career of Pain

Many people, including doctors, find it impossible that someone could have pain over a period of years if he or she really wanted to get rid of it. For a very small number of people (such as Anthony T.), pain does become a career of sorts; pain becomes their chief concern and interest and feeds certain underlying needs they may have no other way of expressing. This route is available to both men and women, but here again the opposite sexes take opposite paths. For a woman to become a career invalid is to take on a classically feminine (in the old sense) role: the bedridden, helpless woman is still "acceptable" in our culture, which continues to see women as fundamentally weak and dependent. For a man to choose this kind of life is to *reject* the traditional male role. Both men and women who opt for invalidism as a way of life are rebelling in a sense, but because the choice has different meanings for each sex, it requires careful interpretation by the individuals involved as well as their friends and family.

A woman who is bored and unchallenged in her life and

who has received little validation of her talents from the world around her may, if she is injured or becomes ill, be drawn to the invalid role because it offers her the personhood she has not found elsewhere. (This role is always there, lurking in the background for any woman who has chronic pain.) Sometimes being incapacitated is, or seems to be, the only way for a woman who has spent a lifetime giving to others and ministering to their needs to receive attention for herself. Her conditioning to be selfless and self-sacrificing may be so powerful that she has no other way of being noticed; disability thus becomes a cry for visibility.

The man who assumes the life of an invalid may be expressing his dissatisfaction with the demands placed upon him to be out in the world and achieving twenty-four hours a day; to be constantly getting ahead, whatever his field of work may be. Despite the past decade's shift in expectations for women, the pressures on men have remained much the same. Even with a working wife, a man is still cast as the one who is out there competing, the living descendant of his hunter forebears. With the additional pressures of rising unemployment and inflation and the increasing cost of the advanced training needed for the higher-paying, more challenging jobs, it is hardly surprising that some men take a long ride on the wave of relief that can accompany an injury or illness that keeps them out of work.

It is important to remember that no one consciously becomes ill or gets hurt in order to receive attention or withdraw from a harsh reality. These common needs can, however, prolong an illness or give texture to its duration if a person has no other outlets for expressing built-up feelings of boredom, anger, exhaustion, depression, or frustration. Part of taking responsibility for your pain lies in becoming aware of the extent to which such feelings play into *your* pain, and why you have them. Once you are aware of them, you can begin consciously to seek out more positive, non-illness-connected ways of deepening your connection to others and being challenged by the work you do and the personal relationships you make.

Your Cultural and Religious Background

Another key context that is bound to have some bearing on how you feel about your pain is your cultural and religious background. Research in this area is inconclusive, but it does seem to indicate a few broad and quite fascinating differences.

There is always a risk in making sweeping judgments and generalizations about whole cultures. It's important to keep in mind as you read through this section that by recognizing the cultural and religious determinants of your pain, you are not judging them. Nor are you judging the way anyone else handles his or her pain. You are taking responsibility for knowing as specifically as you can how these factors contribute to your experience of pain. Every clue you can trace to its source will help you put yourself back together in a new, less painful way as you move along the path to pain control.

Ethnic Differences

The high pain tolerance of indigenous peoples around the world is legendary, as you will remember from the case of the American nurse whose tolerance was so unusually high after her return from living among the Eskimo. In a more recent study reported in the July 18, 1980, issue of *Science* magazine, Nepalese guides in the Himalayas were tested by a team of American investigators using a new technique that can differentiate between a person's ability to *feel* a given stimulus (in this case, electrical stimulation to the wrist and forearm) and the attitudinal factors that determine when the person calls that sensation "pain." The results showed that the Nepalese and American volunteers who were tested at the same time were equally sensitive to the low-grade shocks they received, but that the Nepalese had higher pain tolerance. Dr. W. Crawford Clark and Dr. Suzanne Bennett Clark, coauthors of the report, concluded that the Nepalese were able to take more pain because they had "higher (more stoical) criteria for reporting pain, probably due to their harsh living conditions and other ethnocultural factors such as religion." This experiment is among the first to demonstrate scientifically that people who feel the same measurable amount and kind of pain can and do respond to it very differently because of different cultural interpretations of their experience. In other words, the question "When is pain pain?" can have different answers in different cultural contexts.

Not all Oriental peoples have the same high pain tolerance as the Nepalese, but they may express themselves differently from Westerners when they are in pain. Sometimes Asians or Asian-Americans are perceived by non-Asians as being impassive in the face of pain. A Japanese-American woman explained the cultural logic behind the Oriental attitude toward pain. What Westerners perceive as impassivity is not a lack of feeling. Rather, any dramatic display of emotion, whether of suffering or of joy, is an affront to the Eastern sense of dignity and beauty. To express one's physical suffering with Western-style groans or sighs would be to disturb the smooth, unrippled surface of the natural order.

One of the best-known investigations of ethnic differences in the experience of chronic pain was conducted by the anthropologist Mark Zborowski in a Veterans Administration hospital in New York City in the early 1950s. In *People in*

Pain, based on his interviews with Irish, Italian, Jewish, and "Old American" (WASP) veterans of three wars, Zborowski makes a number of interesting observations.

First of all, he found that the hospital personnel favored the "Old American," or Anglo-Saxon, tradition, which places a high value on self-control and an attitude of detached rationality in discussing one's medical problems. Members of ethnic groups given to more vocal expression of their pain, primarily Jews and Italians, were viewed by the staff as complainers and overreactors.

Zborowski's interviews bore out the staff's impression that people of "Mediterranean origin" were more demonstrative about their pain. He also observed some subtle differences between Jews and Italians that the hospital staff had not picked up. Jews, he found, were more anxious about the significance of their pain in terms of how it would affect their future, and they were less likely than Italians to be satisfied by painkillers, because they viewed any relief as only temporary. Jews asked more questions of doctors and staff, and their concern about the implications of their health was interpreted by staff as overreaction when gauged against the "Old American" model. Based on his interviews, as well as the impressions of the medical personnel, Zborowski found Italians generally more responsive than Jews to pain medication and more grateful; they were also more vociferous when the pain returned. He concluded that the Italians were more present-oriented, while Jews were future-oriented. Whether this is stereotypic speculation or historical reality remains to be seen.

Irish and "Old American" patients shared a calmer, more understated approach to pain and were regarded as "good" patients by the staff. Zborowski found the Irish more reticent and harder to talk to, as well as more emotional when the interviewing process deepened. Here, too, one has to be careful to view these conclusions as no more than a tentative probe of a touchy area of investigation.

Zborowski is properly cautious in evaluating his findings, because there is naturally much room for individual variation within these "stereotypes." Moreover, it appears from his and other studies that the ethnic characteristics he observed are less pronounced in each successive American-born generation. The "Old American" model eventually becomes the norm for people of every origin. Still, even in my own recent interviews with men and women from a broad range of cultural traditions, I found strong echoes of Zborowski's findings.*

Religion

Most major religions have explicit teachings on pain. Even if you weren't raised in strict adherence to a particular doctrine, or if you have stopped practicing the religion in which you were raised, you may hold certain attitudes toward pain that are derived from one or another of the major faiths.

Christianity is the most direct on the subject, since Christ himself is said to have endured not merely pain but torture to redeem humanity. To believing Christians of all denominations, physical pain is meaningful on two important levels: in and of itself, as an echo of Christ's ordeal, and as a profound, transforming experience, through which the suffering of the body refines and purifies the soul, just as Christ's mortal suffering purified the soul of humankind. Christians who wear the symbol of the Cross are wearing the very

---

* To date, no substantial studies have been done of the attitudes toward pain of blacks, Chicanos, and other Hispanic groups in the United States.

essence of their faith's teachings about pain: that pain can be an avenue toward grace and that it has redemptive value.

As recently as June 1980, the Vatican issued a special encyclical in which the Roman Catholic church reiterated its position on the use of painkillers. Suffering, the Vatican declared, "is in fact a sharing in Christ's Passion and a union with the redeeming sacrifice which he offered in obedience to the Father's will. Therefore, one must not be surprised if some Christians prefer to moderate their use of painkillers in order to accept voluntarily at least a part of their sufferings and thus associate themselves in a conscious way with the sufferings of Christ crucified." (The word *excruciating* comes from the practice of crucifixion, *crux* being the Latin word for "cross.") Without exception the Roman Catholics I interviewed spoke of "offering their suffering up to God," expressing a sense of relief at not being alone in their pain and also the hope that some of it could, through belief, be lifted from their shoulders.

Many Christians see pain as a punishment for past sins. In this view, pain has not only a biological or physical cause, but a moral cause as well. It is a message from God, and must be borne with grace as a sign that the message has been heeded. To believers, Christian martyrs are exemplary not only for their extraordinary deeds, but also for the manner in which they bore their final suffering. Several people I interviewed expressed the view that if they still had pain it was because God was not satisfied with the way they were bearing it.

Judaism views pain quite differently. First of all, there is no one Jewish view of pain. Pain itself has no intrinsic meaning within the Jewish religion. It is most often viewed as a random, arbitrary curse whose meaning must be determined by the sufferer. As far back as the Book of Job, which was written more than two thousand years ago, the meaning and place of suffering in a God-created world have been the source of endless questioning for generations of rabbis and scholars. Within the Book of Job itself, several possibilities are at odds: while Job insists on his purity of soul, some of his friends suggest that perhaps he is being punished for some hidden wrongdoing; they urge him to search his conscience for any transgression he has unwittingly committed. In the end, Job never really learns *why* he was made to suffer; but he has kept his faith in God — and this, according to many Jews, is the true meaning of the book. Another interpretation is that Job, in all respects a model Jew and "righteous" man, had to suffer in order to appreciate the power and wondrousness of God: "I have heard of thee by the hearing of the ear: but now mine eye seeth thee."

Unlike the Christian, who can presumably trace pain to a specific sin or wrong attitude, the Jew, like Job, is bewildered. "Why me?" is a typical Jewish response to suffering. Where a believing Christian may assume that God has a reason for sending pain, the Jew isn't sure how pain could be God's work. Perhaps this is the reasoning behind one man's statement to me that he's never *asked* God to take away his pain: "You don't ask for something like that — you pray!" The late Rabbi Milton Steinberg sums up Judaism's views on suffering with these words: "Throughout, it is almost as though Judaism were saying . . . 'By all means strive after insight into this mystery, and may God's favor attend your quest; but never permit yourselves to forget that a *practical* approach to the problem is always before you; that you have it in your power to eliminate many, perhaps most, of the ills that afflict men.'"

Most Eastern religions consider pain an ephemeral experience, because the body itself is seen as belonging to the world of appearance. Only the mind, or soul, is real. Pain, like all bodily feelings, can be transcended. If pain has any meaning, it is as a guide to spiritual evolution. In that sense the believer might welcome pain, but no more than any other experience. The deeply religious Easterner sees all of life as a spiritual journey; pain is no worse and no better than any other experience that comes our way. It is all, in the words of the American guru Baba Ram Dass, "grist for the mill." The German philosopher Eugen Herrigel, who was a lifelong student of Zen Buddhism, explains what acceptance of suffering means in the Oriental context: "Salvation lies in giving full assent to [his] fate, serenely accepting what is laid upon him without asking why he should be singled out for so much suffering. Whoever is able to bear suffering in this way grows to the stature of his suffering, and he detaches himself from it by learning more and more to disregard the fact that it is *his* suffering."

The Economics of Pain

Worlds away from spiritual ruminations on the meaning of suffering are the practical contexts in which pain is lived out day by day. Almost any major illness or injury translates into an extended period of complete or partial unemployment, leaving behind a stack of bills that can literally take years to pay off. But what people who have not experienced chronic pain at close range fail to realize is that chronic pain, whatever its cause, is different from a finite episode of bad health. With chronic pain the bills and increased expenses *continue* to pile up, creating an ongoing drain on your pocketbook, your energy, and your self-esteem. You don't return to work as good as new in a month or take on some extra work to make up for lost time and money. That little push to break you out of debt may be just enough to send you back to bed (or back into traction) again.

Unless you were very well off to begin with, chronic pain will draw you swiftly into the swirl of a vicious economic circle. Suddenly you either are unable to work at all or are working at reduced capacity. Your paid "sick days" evaporate before you even understand what is happening to you. As your income plummets, your expenses soar. The vicious circle looks like this:

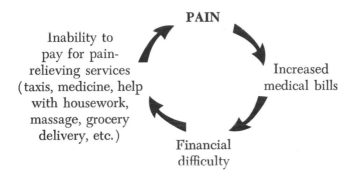

PAIN

Increased
medical bills

Financial
difficulty

Inability to
pay for pain-
relieving services
(taxis, medicine, help
with housework,
massage, grocery
delivery, etc.)

The economic consequences of pain to society as a whole have been calculated in figures so astronomical they practically defy comprehension. According to Dr. David Bresler, director of the U.C.L.A. Pain Control Unit, $50 billion annually is spent in this country for pain-related disability and medical services. Low back pain alone, according to the National Center for Health Statistics, accounts for 18 million doctor visits a year in the United States and is the leading cause of disability in most Western countries. The National Arthritis Foundation quotes the figure of $8 billion a year in lost wages and disability; patients, the foundation says, spend another $4 billion a year on various forms of medical care — all these billions just for arthritis. How do these staggering figures translate in individual terms?

In addition to the strictly medical expenses of chronic pain (doctor visits, hospitalizations, various treatments including physical therapy and medication), only some of which are covered by most insurance policies, there is also a whole range of extra expenses for which no coverage exists. There is the cost of moving and the higher rent of an apartment in an elevator building if one can no longer climb stairs. Taxis, once a luxury, become a necessity in cities where mass transit is made difficult by lack of benches, steep stairways, and longer waits between trains and buses due to budget cutbacks. I found that a whole range of everyday activities suddenly acquired a price tag after I got sick. Grocery shopping in supermarkets, for example, with their endless aisles and long checkout lines, exacerbated my pain beyond what I could take. I found that I needed either to do one large shopping trip every couple of weeks, which meant laying out a lot of money all at once and paying for delivery, or else to patronize the smaller shops closer to home, where prices were higher. Either way, I was spending a great deal more for food than I had before, even taking inflation into account.

Sometimes being in pain can force you to forego simple forms of recreation that might play a major role in alleviating your sense of isolation and tension. Going to a movie or a sports event may be within your budget, but if you are unable to make the trip by public transportation, you may have to draw the line at the ten- or twenty-dollar round-trip taxi fare to get you there and back.

Another serious hardship I have encountered is the increasing practice among doctors and other health professionals of requiring payment immediately after services are rendered — before you even leave their office. How often have I wanted to launch into a diatribe about how that thirty-five or fifty dollars was just the money I needed to eat with!

When you're in pain and broke, or close to broke, you're at one of life's all-time low points, where the vicious economic circle interlocks with another vicious circle: the circle of despair.

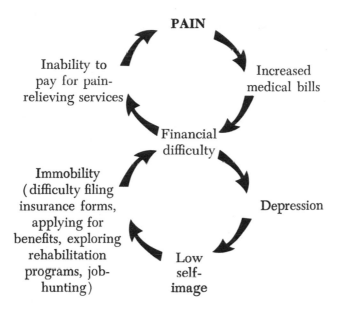

PAIN

Inability to
pay for pain-
relieving services

Increased
medical bills

Financial
difficulty

Immobility
(difficulty filing
insurance forms,
applying for
benefits, exploring
rehabilitation
programs, job-
hunting)

Depression

Low
self-
image

The Way Out

No matter how difficult matters get, it is essential not to let
yourself get stuck in either/or choices. There are always
new ways of accomplishing your goals if the old ones are
no longer feasible. Even when your financial resources are
extremely limited, you *can* turn the tide. It takes energy, ingenuity and, above all, the knowledge that you are not alone.
Our health care system doesn't make it easy for you, and as
of this writing it looks as though we can expect hard times
ahead. The first step is to take responsibility for seeing to it
that you are getting the best mileage out of all the currently
available programs (see the Coping Resource Guide on pages
231–42 for concrete suggestions on where to get advice).

The second step is to apply your problem-solving skills
and ingenuity to your vocational situation. Being in pain
forces you to use your imagination and peer around the
obstacles on your path to discover what lies beyond. By

carefully, calmly, and intelligently analyzing all your abilities, past, present, and potential, you can get back on the track and thrive again as a productive person. An excellent book to read in this regard is Richard Nelson Bolles's beautifully assembled job counseling manual, *What Color Is Your Parachute?* I recommend it highly for its sound advice, entertaining format, and extensive reference section.

The third step is to fight back by organizing with other people in the same situation to ensure that your common interests lead to necessary changes in our health care delivery system. A number of groups representing a broad range of interests are working around the country to create information networks and alternative health care centers and to bring about legal and structural changes at the highest levels of government. You'll find a partial listing in the Coping Resource Guide on pages 231–42.

Meanwhile, you may want to review the list below as you sort out your economic situation and take stock of your immediate options.

- Be sure that you are getting the most out of your current insurance plan; reread your policy or call a representative of your insurance company. If you are receiving Medicaid, a staff person in your local Medicaid office should be able to explain the full range of benefits to you.

- Investigate all sources of aid — federal, state, city, and neighborhood — for which you may be eligible.

- If you are unable to work at the job for which you were trained, find out about vocational rehabilitation programs near where you live. Check under "Office of Vocational Rehabilitation" or "Department of Rehabilitation" in your local telephone directory.

- Explore the possibility of supplementing your present income by putting your existing talents to use. You may be able to work at home and find a local market for what you make, bake, or grow.

- Pool your resources with others to create shortcuts around some of the obstacles on your path. You may be able to arrange rides to shopping centers, borrow or trade books, and so on.

- Know your community and use it. Whether you're involved with a religious group, an extended family, a senior citizens' center, a political organization, or the women's movement, by reaching out to the network of people in which *you* feel a sense of belonging, you will find both moral support and a rewarding way of remaining connected.

Age

Your age is another important context that shapes your experience of pain. Even more than your actual chronological age, how you feel about your age can have a decisive impact on your pain. Almost everyone I interviewed referred indirectly to age by saying, "This is a hell of a time for me to have ———" (whatever their condition was). For Hannah, who at seventy-four felt she had earned the right to a measure of serenity after a lifetime of hard work, the worsening of her arthritis was a harsh accompaniment to the so-called golden years. Rosalie, injured at twenty-five, felt the injustice of pain marring her "best years" and hampering her efforts to strike out on her own in a new city and to form a lasting relationship. Paul, thirty-five and in the "prime of life," was bitter at having health problems that made him feel prematurely old.

Perhaps Edna summed it up best when she said simply, "I wasn't ready." No one is ever ready for pain. There is no "good" time for it. Assuming it were desirable to learn ahead of time to deal with pain (as some people are now advocating), all the preparation in the world would still leave people in pain feeling, "I wasn't ready. Couldn't it have happened at a better time?"

The main way age interacts with pain is in our perception that both age and pain are inevitable once they "set in." This fossilized outlook afflicts both young and old alike, but it is particularly debilitating for the old. The older people I interviewed tended to be far more pessimistic about doing anything to modify or mitigate their pain: "At my age you can't expect miracles" was a typical response. With such an outlook, any affliction appears as a confirmation of the time-worn belief that old age is a sickness. The great French writer Colette, bedridden with arthritis in the final decade of her life, had a very different view of pain. "Pain," she wrote, nearing eighty, "that sharp recall to life!"

In the past ten years, older people have begun to challenge many of the stereotypes about age and aging. As one extraordinary woman told me, you are always growing, always evolving. The way an older person responds to pain, she said, depends on how he or she learned to meet prior challenges in life. Because the aging, by the very fact of their survival, have lost many of their support systems — jobs, friends, spouses, family members, neighbors known for years — she emphasized the importance of making a special effort to combat the loneliness and isolation many people face as they get old. "Social vitamins," in her words, are as important as nutritional meals for staying vital even in pain. This woman found her "social vitamins" by becoming politically active on behalf of older Americans and improved health care.

For those like Paul and Rosalie who feel prematurely old, it is important to undo the shorthand thinking that links pain and disability with age. Just as that connection can lead older people to despair and resignation, it can have the same effect on us. One way of looking at pain is to consider it an extra complication, but by no means the only one, we have to deal with right now in our life. With or without pain, if you are young you have one set of issues to deal with, and if you are middle-aged or old you have another. No matter how old you are, even if your underlying medical condition can't be substantially changed, and even though you can't roll back the clock, you can apply every single one of the suggestions in this book. So long as your mind is open to learning, you can learn to cope with pain.

Your Living Arrangements

As important a context as your age and your economic situation is your current living arrangement, both in terms of personal relationships to friends or loved ones and in terms of the actual physical surroundings in which you live. In Chapter 11, "Pain-Free Relating," we'll take a closer look at how your spouse or lover, friends, and others are — and can best be — involved in your experience of pain. For the moment let it suffice to take note of the kinds of social connections you currently have, how satisfied (or dissatisfied) you are with your present friendships and love relationships, and whom you can count on in hard times and who can count on you.

If you have close, important friendships or a warm home life, you have precious sources not only of support and understanding but of excitement, company, and, so important and so often underestimated, opportunities for getting out of yourself and giving to others. If your current living arrangements are a source of unhappiness, this is certainly an area that needs further reflection.

Sometimes a minute, seemingly insignificant gesture can have enormous consequences. If you've ever sailed, you know the kind of geometric increase you get from pushing the tiller an inch or two and sending the boat in a whole new direction. By learning to think in terms of increments (instead of imagining vast projects that might take years to bring to fruition), you may find that you can bring about astonishing and even exhilarating changes in your life with the smallest acts of your imagination. A phone call can set a new friendship in motion. When it comes to your physical surroundings, you may find inspiration in the kind of ingenuity that was second nature to Colette:

> Certainly it is a pleasure to lie facing a spectacle of lights and shades without so much as having to raise oneself on an elbow, without craning one's neck or sitting up in bed, and never to take one's eyes off it till the curtain of their lids is lowered. Whatever is easily come by is always a pleasure, even when distilled by a drop of bitterness: if I did not suffer ... this ... well, this agony, I should never have thought of positioning my bed, calculated to a nicety, in the corner where its occupant is afforded an untrammeled view of three horizons.

"Any point of change changes all your horizons," one older woman told me. If this is the wisdom that comes with age, let us honor it as we turn to Chapter 6 where the art of listening becomes the key to change.

6

Learning to Listen:
Your Pain May Be Trying
to Tell You Something

Illness is the doctor to whom we pay most heed. To kindness, to knowledge, we make promises only; pain we obey.

MARCEL PROUST

"Dr. Abernethy," said a patient, "I have something the matter, Sir, with this arm. There, oh! (making a particular motion with the limb) That, Sir, gives me great pain."
"Well, what a fool you must be to do it then," said Dr. Abernethy.

The Memoirs of
John Abernethy (1764–1831)

Proust was right: pain exacts obedience. But obedience has many modes and many meanings, ranging from complete submission to grudging compliance to creative responsiveness. You now have the self-knowledge that can lead to

93

creative responsiveness, which is not only the most rewarding but by far the healthiest form of obedience to pain. By learning to listen to your pain, you will begin to practice the creative obedience that grows out of knowledge and into pain control.

Finding the right balance between noticing and not noticing pain is one of the trickiest aspects of learning to live with chronic pain. It is a well-known fact that if you can limit yourself when you first feel pain, you have a lot more freedom later on. This is easily said and harder done. Most people have a tendency to swing back and forth between ignoring their pain for as long as they can and then collapsing, between overextending themselves and overlimiting themselves. By learning to listen to your pain from the beginning, you can avoid all these unnecessary swings between too much and too little. Instead of being painfully aware of your limitations, you can use your awareness of pain to extend your limits to the very edge of possibility. The image I like to keep in mind is of learning to live at the end of my rope — not the frayed, taut rope of exhaustion, but the flexible, ever-lengthening rope that follows the path to pain control.

Pain Is a Loud Message

Pain is a loud message. It hurts, and if we ignore it, it gets louder and louder until we are forced to pay attention. By putting off our response we run the risk that the underlying physical process can become exacerbated and end up requiring more attention than it would have if we had responded quickly and responsibly in the first place.

Strangely enough, the way you respond to the morning alarm may give you some very interesting insights into the way you react to the loud message of pain. When this idea first dawned on me, I realized that in both pain and sleep I was playing at seeing how far I could go before I was forced to give in. My morning ritual involves setting the alarm to ring at least an hour before I need to be up and then resetting it at fifteen-minute intervals until I absolutely have to get out of bed. Given my personality this makes sense, because in general I thrive on risks. But when I thought about it in relation to pain, it made no sense at all. All I was doing was hurting myself. I now make a conscious effort to respond to my pain before matters get out of hand. With pain even more than with sleep, it's important to hear the alarm and begin responding to it right away. This first level of reacting to pain is primarily one of logistics. It involves the simple, step-by-step decisions that can make all the difference in how much pain you have at the end of the day.

Migraine headaches are known for the warning "auras" they give off. Many people have learned to head off the agonies of full-blown migraine by following a few simple steps (darkening a room, practicing a form of relaxation such as meditation or the relaxation response, lying down in a quiet place) as soon as they feel the first signs of an attack. Many other chronic conditions also give warnings before they escalate into severe pain. With certain muscular and neuromuscular conditions, feelings of fatigue or achiness precede actual pain and are a clear sign that the body needs some form of rest. For some people, just sitting down for a few minutes can be enough to prevent painful muscle spasms; for others, elevating the legs, applying cold packs, or taking a warm bath may be more appropriate. In almost every conceivable pain situation it pays to listen right from the start and begin responding right away, based on what your pain needs at that moment. It's just like answering the questions in the back of your mind; the faster you respond, the less chance the pain compounders have of getting under your skin.

In order to respond most fully to your pain, you need to develop the fine-tuning of your inner ear so you can "hear" exactly what your pain is asking for. That's why the concept that completes the three R's of pain control is *receptivity*, the art of listening.

What Is Receptivity?

Insects have antennae to pick up distant signals of danger and to help them orient themselves in the world. They cannot hear, but their antennae allow them to feel. Radios have antennae to pick up signals from distant transmitters. Human beings have no antennae; instead, we have the mental and emotional sensitivity to be highly aware of what is happening around us as well as within us. Just as we sometimes need to fine-tune a radio to get the clearest reception, there are times when we need to sharpen our own reception.

Receptivity is both a mental attitude and a specific set of skills. Being receptive means being open to receiving. This is by no means a passive concept. Rather, it is an attitude that conveys a willingness to go out and find what *you* need in order to feel less pain. Being receptive means being open to modes of thought that might be helpful, useful, and exciting; to new methods of coping with pain that you may have heard of but not actually tried; and to the world around you, strengthening your connections to the people, ideas, and activities you already care about as well as forming new ones. Receptivity is a way of coping that honors you as a person by respecting the many different factors that make your pain unique.

The exercises that follow are based on the multifaceted

expertise you have acquired in the preceding chapters. They have been designed to help you receive the clearest signals possible from your pain and to fine-tune your responses for maximum effect. By developing the art of receptivity you will learn to detect your pain sooner and obey it faster and more constructively. The pain control you will come to master, beginning in this chapter, is the creative obedience the theologian Alan Watts meant when he wrote of "controlling ourselves by cooperating with ourselves."

What Is Your Body Asking For?

Animals don't create blocking mechanisms for ignoring pain. They already know how to listen. As Dr. James F. Fries points out in *Arthritis: A Comprehensive Guide*, "Animals do very well with arthritis and muscle problems because they let that internal doctor — pain — guide their activities." We humans have to retrain ourselves to hear exactly what our internal doctor is trying to tell us. Civilization has progressively divorced us from our animal siblings, mostly by splitting our minds from our bodies and leaving us in a perilous state of detachment from our physical selves. Those of us working and living in today's technologically advanced postindustrial societies often have painstakingly to relearn, in workshops and even college courses, the rudimentary bodily awareness that was instinctive for our ancestors. Very few of us are as in tune with our bodies as Nancy, the marathon runner, who told me, "The pain is my barometer. I can tell just by the pain where I am."

Bodily awareness is a crucial part of coping with pain, because besides pain you may be feeling all sorts of other sensations that can give you valuable signals for pain control. For example, a number of people I interviewed observed that when they are in pain they get very hungry;

some need sugar; others get very tired and need extra sleep. If you fine-tune your awareness you may notice that besides the sensation of pain (which clamors the loudest but is never alone), you are feeling cold, a bodily "need" that can usually be dealt with simply and quickly by putting on a sweater or closing an open window. By responding to such sensations as temperature or hunger you can indirectly have a positive effect on your overall sense of well-being, which in turn will positively affect your pain. The first step in learning to listen is learning to take a simple inventory whenever you begin to feel pain. In addition to helping you focus on what you can do for your pain, the Fast Check on page 99 opens you up to your surroundings, setting the stage for enhanced receptivity.

Practice Makes Perfect

Learning to listen to what your pain is saying takes practice. If your pain is chronic, you have ample opportunity — you might even want to start today. Remember, no matter what the situation, even if you are at work and under pressure or on a strict schedule, you *always* have choices. You *can* tip the balance. Just because you can't take a hot bath in your office at two o'clock in the afternoon doesn't mean there aren't other steps that will reduce your pain. It's up to you to find the right steps for each situation. You have all the know-how that you need.

Which Way Do You Tip the Balance?

Read through the reports from Rosalie, Paul, and the others on the following pages. Then go back to the Pain Inventory you filled out on page 61. Put yourself in a situation in which

Fast Check

Each time you run through the following inventory in your mind you will learn something new, because your pain skills are constantly developing. Right this second, as you are reading these words, try to get in touch with everything you are feeling in your body. Focus in as fast as you can, filling in the appropriate spaces with a few key words.

Today's Date _____ Pain Level (see page 34) _____

Where am I? _____ What time is it? _____

Is this where I usually am at this time or is this an unusual place for me to be? _____

If I look up from this page, what are the first three things I see?

What am I aware of in my body?

1. _____

☐ Hunger

2. _____

☐ Thirst

3. _____

☐ Fatigue

What can I hear?

☐ Tension

☐ Sexual feelings

☐ Pain

Am I:

What can I smell?

☐ Cold?

☐ Hot?

☐ Just right?

If I am in pain, what are three things I could try right away that might help?

1. _____

2. _____

3. _____

you are frequently in pain. You may want to use the 10 A.M. self-portrait from page 38, but feel free to vary it with any other setting, provided you choose a situation drawn from your personal experience. As you did in your Self-Portrait back on page 36, in the space provided describe your situation succinctly. Where are you; why are you there; what time of day is it; what are you doing? Give your pain level based on the Plain Ordinary Pain Scale on page 34. Imagine the factors that would *increase* your pain in this particular situation. List them. Then list the factors that might *decrease* your pain. You have the power to tip the balance either way. Which way do you ordinarily tip the balance in the situation you have described?

Rosalie   6

It's five o'clock on a Tuesday afternoon. I'm at work. By this time of day I have shooting pains up and down both of my legs. My back is really throbbing. After the accident I took a room right around the corner from my job, so I don't have far to walk; but I still find it hard to get up and leave the office. I'm in too much pain to shop or cook, and I can't afford to eat out. I wish I had some place else to go besides back to my room. I hardly know anyone here, because the accident happened three weeks after I arrived.

Could increase my pain: standing, walking, sitting, hunger, loneliness

Could decrease my pain: warm bath, lying in bed, painting, relaxing, friends

Which way do I tip the balance? Toward decreasing pain, but could do more.

Paul   0

It's eleven o'clock on a Saturday morning. I slept late, because I don't usually work on the weekend unless I have to. But when I'm not working I'm sort of at loose ends. Financially I'm way behind from the time I was in the hospital, so I'm constantly feeling I should be doing extra work. But I don't feel like pushing myself too hard. My place is a real mess. I should really clean it up so I can set up my darkroom. Every Saturday I think about doing it, but I'm afraid of throwing my back out again.

Could increase my pain: lifting heavy objects, worrying, feeling depressed

Could decrease my pain: taking it easy, not sure what else

Which way do I tip the balance? Toward pain.

Edna   10

It's ten A.M. I'm sitting at the kitchen table staring out the window. I'm alone in the house. Mornings are my worst time because the whole day is still ahead. I think about my old job and what they're doing right now. Then I feel real bad. I can't do anything anymore, not even the shopping. My husband has to do the cooking. I envy my friends because they're not in pain, but I know that's a sinful attitude. I feel guilty that people from church still come to visit me. I don't deserve it. I have no way of paying them back.

Could increase my pain: standing, walking, lifting heavy objects, worrying

Could decrease my pain: ice packs, lying down, not sure what else

Which way do I tip the balance? Toward pain.

Frank   6

It's one o'clock on a Monday afternoon. I just got back to my desk from my lunch break. This morning I saw four kids, and now my hands feel too stiff and achy to write any more reports. But I have another three appointments this afternoon, and then a meeting with the two other psychologists from my division after school. When I have the whole afternoon ahead of me I always have a sort of clutched feeling, because I know the pain's going to get worse and worse.

Could increase my pain: writing, worrying
Could decrease my pain: writing less, relaxing, heating pad, ointment
Which way do I tip the balance? Increase pain.

Jack   6

It's three o'clock on a Sunday afternoon and all my in-laws are over. My wife's father is eighty-five and he doesn't see very well so I have to help him every time he wants to get up for something. We're a very close family and we've been having him over once a week for the past thirty years; it means a lot to my wife. But I really take a beating being the host. We always end up making a barbecue out in back in the warmer months, because it's nice for the kids and we can all use a little sunshine. By the end I can't wait for them all to leave so I can collapse on the sofa.

Could increase my pain: walking, lifting, carrying, tension
Could decrease my pain: lying down, reading the paper, smoking a pipe
Which way do I tip the balance? Increase pain.

Hannah   10

It's three o'clock on a weekday afternoon. You wouldn't think at my age time could go so slowly. But from now until I go to bed I have only pain to look forward to. And even then it's not as if I get any respite. It's really torture. I used to look forward to going out in the evening, especially to concerts. Now I'm stuck. It takes me ten minutes just to go from the living room to the dining room! Arthritis is a cage. Right now I feel like steel spikes are going into me. I try to sit as still as I can, but even when I don't move the pain is unbelievable.

Could increase my pain: moving or staying still — everything increases it

Could decrease my pain: nothing

Which way do I tip the balance? I have no choice.

It's

Could increase my pain:

Could decrease my pain:

Which way do I tip the balance?

Replay

In this replay of the situation you have just described, you and the others get a second chance. This time, imagine yourself taking all the steps that could lead to pain reduction — or at least to keeping your pain at its present level. Be guided by your internal doctor as you put the art of receptivity into practice.

Rosalie
It's five o'clock on a Tuesday afternoon. A friend of mine is meeting me downstairs when I get out of work, and we're going to pick up some sandwiches and go back to my place to eat. I don't know her very well,

but I decided to give her a call. I'd like to know her better. She knows I was hurt, and I told her I can't walk very far after working all day. But maybe our friendship will grow, and that would be nice. She'll be my first guest in my new room!

Paul

It's eleven o'clock on a Saturday morning. I'm going to start fixing up my place. I figured out a way to start setting things up for the darkroom without hurting my back. I'm going to give myself a month, four Saturdays in a row. I'm under a lot of pressure because of my debts, but it's true I need to get back my old sense of myself as somebody able to enjoy life and pursue my photography, which I do care about. So I'll do this in a nonpressured way, and try not to think about money while I'm cleaning. I'll listen to music.

Edna

It's ten A.M. I'm going to call the two women who are supposed to come visit me this afternoon from our parish, and tell them I think it would be a nice day for us to go to the park across the street. Maybe if I got out of the house once in a while I wouldn't feel so weak. We don't have any folding chairs, but maybe one of them could bring one. I think I'll also ask them if there's any way I can get a ride to their weekly meetings. I guess there's no medical reason why I shouldn't go. After I make the phone call I'm going to lie down with an ice pack on my neck so I'll be more relaxed when they come.

Frank

It's one o'clock on a Monday afternoon. I just got back to my desk from my lunch break and another kid is due for an interview in a few minutes. I'm going to put some of that terrific new Chinese ointment on my hands and wrap them in a heating pad. Since my hands are so stiff, I think I'll record the afternoon interviews on cassettes and try to write them up tonight at home. I have to find out about whether I'm entitled to use the school's secretarial staff for occasional typing. Maybe I can work something out.

Jack
It's three o'clock on a Sunday afternoon and all my in-laws are over. After all these years it finally dawned on me that there are enough other people in the family for me to take it easy. My sons are big boys now, so they can watch out for their grandfather. I'm sitting on a chaise lounge in the back yard. I made drinks for everyone because at least that much I can do. Now I've got my legs up and I'm out in the sun enjoying myself. The pain is still there but I'm not really thinking about it.

Hannah
It's three o'clock on a weekday afternoon. I'm listening to a beautiful string quartet on the radio and waiting for my physical therapist to arrive. My daughter found out about a program where they come twice a week to your house and teach you some exercises and help you take a bath. So far there haven't been any miracles, but the therapist says at least now I have a chance of keeping a little mobility. Also, the exercises in the bathtub are very relaxing. She works with a lady a few blocks from here who used to be a violinist, and she wants us to meet. She said she'll help us get together.

It's

I am still learning to listen. I still do replays in my mind. But by now I have a feeling for when I am "betraying" myself by pushing too hard or by ignoring my body's clear signals. Sometimes I consciously choose to ignore my body's loud call for rest because there is something I want so badly to do that I am willing to take the consequences. When I make such a choice, I almost automatically visualize in my mind's eye exactly what I am going to do afterwards to minimize my pain. If I go to a movie and I'm already in level 2 or 3 pain, I will probably not stay out very late, which would intensify the pain, or walk more than a few steps afterwards to a café. Chances are I'd take a nice hot bath before climbing into bed. There are still times when I slip up, but I know that each day is part of the learning process — part of my own path to pain control.

As you learn to listen, you learn the full extent of what is possible for you. Sometimes you may have to hold back on what you do. But most of the time you can do a lot more than you may have realized.

Listening for the Possible

Once you have learned to heed the cues and clues your body provides by taking immediate measures to ease your pain, you can begin to move toward a more far-reaching kind of receptivity. This sort of thinking involves developing your long-range antennae so that you are able to live the fullest, most productive life you can, no matter what your physical condition is.

All of us experience moments of painlessness from time to time. An upsetting phone call can momentarily distract your attention from your pain. So can more positive involvements, such as hearing a stirring speech about something you believe in, or putting your kids to sleep with their favorite bedtime story and sharing their delight. Actually, such moments occur throughout the day. These moments of pain-lessness are like little chinks of light that let us glimpse a life beyond pain. Training yourself to notice them extends the art of receptivity to heighten your awareness of the specific activities that bring you the greatest freedom from pain.

For some, satisfaction lies in skills or crafts that test their ingenuity and provide a tangible outlet for their creativity; for others, nothing is more pleasant than a good novel or the pursuit of lifelong interests by reading works of nonfiction. For still others, active involvement in any number of local groups can provide both temporary freedom from pain and a sense of enduring commitment to the well-being of others. Being in pain doesn't prevent you from learning or giving. Almost anything you are deeply involved in can lead to long periods of painlessness.

When you become truly absorbed in any activity, whether work or play, you simply can't feel as much pain as you do when you are sitting around doing nothing but suffering. Your body doesn't have enough circuits to process that much information at one time, and it wisely chooses to record pleasure over pain.* This is why it is so important to be aware of every single activity you could be doing and every way you can be active, both physically *and* mentally. The more you *use* yourself, the less pain you will feel.

You may have to make a conscious effort to think of yourself as someone who can instead of someone who can't. Pain often causes us to shrink from doing things that might give us great pleasure, because we are afraid of exacerbating our pain. When holding back becomes a reflex action, as it so easily can, you may be ruling out activities you are perfectly

---

* According to Dr. John G. Hannington-Kiff, the mechanism of this effect "is probably that the central nervous system ceases to evaluate noxious stimuli as pain when it is otherwise engaged in *pursuits of greater current relevance to the life of the individual*" (italics mine).

capable of doing with little or no risk of increasing your pain. It is also common to get stuck in a sense of loss over what you can no longer do. This period of grief is a natural part of the chronic pain process, but it is also natural and necessary to look beyond what you can't do to what you *can* do.

Listing the Possible

The following exercise involves three lists. The first is a list of all the activities your pain actually prevents you from pursuing. Include hobbies and special interests, as well as vocational skills and everyday activities such as lifting heavy objects, getting in and out of a bathtub, driving, or combing your hair. The second is a list of all the activities you have stopped doing because of your pain, but that you might actually be able to do — perhaps with some modification or help. List 3 has space for activities you don't ordinarily do — some that you may never even have tried — but that you may now have the time and inclination to pursue.

1. Can No Longer Do	2. Could Be Doing	3. New Activities
1.	1.	1.
2.	2.	2.
3.	3.	3.
4.	4.	4.
5.	5.	5.
6.	6.	6.
7.	7.	7.
8.	8.	8.
9.	9.	9.
10.	10.	10.

Look back over your lists, with special attention to List 1. Can you say exactly why each of the activities you listed is impossible for you now? Are you sure there aren't a few that couldn't be nudged over into List 2? Be sure you use your imagination here; there may be certain activities you can no longer do as easily or alone but that you could do with assistance or modification.

> The life-force may be the least understood force on earth. William James said that human beings tend to live too far within self-imposed limits. It is possible that these limits will recede when we respect more fully the natural drive of the human mind and body toward perfectibility and regeneration. Protecting and cherishing that natural drive may well represent the finest exercise of human freedom.
>
> NORMAN COUSINS

The Importance of Taking Risks

The goal of learning to listen and of all these exercises is to help you figure out a way to keep lengthening your rope. You want to be able to have less pain not by learning to sit still and do nothing, but while extending your sense of the possible to encompass a range of satisfying and productive activities. Pain itself never sits still; it is constantly changing. So part of the process of learning to live with it involves taking risks — those small stretches without which you will never find out just how far you can go. To me, risks are the spice of life. However, with pain you want to go easy. It's important to take your risks with care.

I remember planning a research trip to Washington, D.C. I was in a lot of pain and began to wonder if I should go after all. Just getting from my house to the train station was going to be hard, so how was I going to be after a four-hour jounce on the New York–Washington rails? And then what? Getting to a place to stay? I began to envision trouble. I decided maybe I should put off my trip until I was feeling a little stronger on my feet. After all, how much work would I get done in Washington if I was having trouble concentrating on my work in New York? Then I had a conversation with myself. I decided that I would go ahead with the trip, planning it in such a way that I would have safety nets all along the way. I had friends in Philadelphia and Baltimore, the two main stops between New York and Washington. By making a daylong stopover in Philadelphia I accomplished three things: I saw dear friends, I gave my body a chance to rest thoroughly before getting back on the train again, and I had a chance to stop and reevaluate my plans at a distance from which I could more easily return to New York if it proved necessary. I also cut my stay in Washington from four days to two, to minimize the wear and tear on my legs. The end result of all this careful planning was that I went farther away from my house than I had in a whole year, wound up in a lot of pain, but returned home satisfied with what I had accomplished. It was a risk, but by breaking it into small pieces I was able to go through with it. I also learned that travel really *is* a risk for me and that it's not something I can contemplate with enthusiasm.

Risks don't have to take you far afield. Just inviting friends to dinner when you're feeling awful can also be a risk. Company may keep you connected to people you love — and cheer you or distract you but not if you insist on being the ultimate host or hostess and doing everything yourself when you're in pain. For me, the risk in entertaining lies in learning to sit still — or relatively still — and letting other people jump up and down: a real challenge to my hale self-image. You have to keep trying things, or you'll never know how long your rope can be. With chronic pain, small risks take you a lot further than big ones. If you push yourself to the point of masochism, you end up making your pain much worse. That doesn't lengthen your rope; it yanks you back against the wall.

Keeping a Pain Journal

Each time you face a different situation in pain, you have the opportunity to try your listening and risking skills anew. I'm sure you'll find, as I did, that over the weeks and months you become surer and surer of yourself as you see the ideas and exercises in this book begin to make a real difference in your day-to-day life.

One excellent way of keeping track of your progress and actually speeding yourself along the path to pain control is to keep a Pain Journal. A plain ruled notebook of any size makes a perfect journal. A fairly small one is especially practical for carrying around. My own journal goes with me wherever I go, and it has taught me more than I would ever have imagined. Even if you only keep it on a daily basis for a week or two, a journal can give you an invaluable sense not only of the fluctuations in your pain, but also of the kinds of situations you find most difficult and the techniques that work best for you. Most important of all, a Pain Journal allows you to express some of your private feelings about pain and to think out creative solutions. There is no better way of learning to listen.

The sample entry on page 112 will show you how easy it is to get started. Some basic guidelines for keeping a Pain Journal:

- Date each entry at the top of the page.
- Use the Plain Ordinary Scale on page 34 to record your pain level each time you write.
- Write freely without censoring yourself, then summarize for easy reference by focusing on the three key topics shown at the bottom of the sample entry: your feelings, conclusions, and plan of action.

Today's Date: September 12, 1978	Pain Level: 4

I woke up feeling really terrible. It's one of those days when the pain's so bad you just want to stay in bed — but I decided to put myself through all my paces and see what would happen. I got out of bed and put on some nice classical music and then I wrapped one of those freezable gels around my neck with a towel. Just to be "safe" I took two aspirin! Now it's 11 o'clock and I don't feel any worse than when I woke up. That's a big improvement compared to yesterday! Everybody's out at work, so I decided to try my luck with the Help Wanted ads and see if there was anything I might be able to do part-time, just to get back to work somewhat. I actually got up the guts to call one place — you don't need any particular experience and I didn't tell them my skills were a little rusty. I didn't even say anything about the accident. So I have an interview tomorrow! Anyway, it's in a hospital, so if I start to fall apart . . . Will keep you posted . . .

My feelings: I feel excited, proud, and optimistic. Also, just for the record, a little cynical. It would be too good to be true.

Conclusions: My new attitude seems to be paying off — trying not to think of myself as someone "sick," someone in pain.

Plan of action: Keep it up!

Up to this point, the emphasis of *The Path to Pain Control* has been on what might be called the Ecology of Pain. By conserving your best energy and using your inner resources — ingenuity, imagination, and plain common sense — you have learned how to reduce your pain to an absolute minimum given your physical condition. No one has to tell you which factors and attitudes alleviate your pain and which ones exacerbate it; you know yourself, and you may have already begun to reap the fruits of your knowledge by practicing the art of listening.

There's a beautiful Zen tale that compares the fates of a slender bamboo shoot and an oak tree in a blizzard. According to the story, the oak tree, mighty and unyielding, breaks under the force of the wind and the weight of the snow. The supple, graceful bamboo stalk bends with the storm and holds its own. Like the oak, we have been trained to stand firm and resist the burdens that come our way. Like the oak, we easily break under the strain. But the skills you have acquired in the preceding chapters have brought you a long way from the oak's unbending might toward the supple strength of the bamboo. You know now that in the storm of chronic pain you have the greatest range of options and the greatest chance of reducing your suffering when, like the wise bamboo, you deal with your pain from the beginning, responding with clarity and responsibility instead of waiting until it has gotten out of hand.

You know now that every moment holds a choice: toward painlessness or toward pain. As you continue to apply the exercises and overall approach of this book, you will become more and more skilled in making the choices that move you toward painlessness and away from pain. New choices establish new patterns. As your "right" choices add up, you will find that you have come a long way indeed on the path to pain control.

You will find, too, that the presence of pain in your life, while certainly not something you would have chosen, can become a life-giving rather than a life-depleting force. You can't choose to have no pain, but you *can* choose to have less pain and to turn your pain energy into life energy — energy that works for you. This is the ultimate challenge of chronic pain, and the one we turn to next.

7

Turning Pain Energy into Life Energy

> Now, if I am lying here motionless tonight, there is good reason for it, for I can feel stirring within me— apart from the twisting pain, as if under the heavy screw of a winepress — a far less constant turnscrew than pain, an insurrection of the spirit.
>
> COLETTE

You now know that it is possible to reach a new and lower level of pain. You know how to get there. At this point a new question appears on the horizon. Once you've begun to make significant strides toward pain control and you're doing everything in your power to keep your pain to a real minimum, how do you cope with the pain that remains? The answer lies in a series of techniques that can help you use your residual pain as a source of energy for getting on with what makes life worth living for you.

The Alchemy of Pain

The alchemists of old believed they could turn ordinary metals into gold. They never did strike gold, but the word survives, a wonderful hybrid that reflects its origin in the medieval laboratories where East met West. *Alchemy* puts Arabic and Greek together to mean "a transformation."

When it comes to chronic pain, the science of alchemy is alive and well. You can transform pain into non-pain through any number of visualization techniques such as those described in the Pain Emergency Kit beginning on page 209. For example, the next time you're in pain you might try thinking of your pain as fine sand running through the area of your body that hurts. This sort of mental "restructuring" of pain can be applied to great advantage in short-term situations including insomnia. When you consciously use pain to create an unexpected, enjoyable experience for yourself, even if that experience lasts only two or three minutes, you are turning pain energy into life energy. This is alchemy made modern — and practical.

Here's another example. Let's say it's two o'clock on a weekday afternoon. Put yourself where you usually are at that time of day. Your pain level is pretty high. What you want right now is simply to put off your usual reaction — whether that's smoking a cigarette, taking a painkiller, clenching your teeth, or complaining to the person closest at hand — in order to try something different for a few minutes. Feel the pain. Feel its energy. Now imagine yourself taking that energy and doing something with it that you wouldn't ordinarily do. It may be something as simple as getting up and looking out the window (whether you're at home or at work). Look at the sky — but really look at it. Notice the tones of blues or grays, the kinds of clouds if there are any, the position of the sun (or lack of it), the pattern of trees or buildings against the horizon. If you're in a place where there's a busy street outside, you might want to spend a few minutes watching the passersby — how they're dressed, how they walk, the expressions on their faces. This is not pure distraction; it is the conscious, deliberate substitution of a pleasurable experience for a painful one. What you are doing is taking the impact of pain — the force with which it seems to invade your body and your life — and choosing to use it for something other than protracted suffering.

One of the true masters of this art was Colette, who met the challenge of life in a wheelchair with characteristic charisma and creativity:

> For anyone not able to dawdle along a pavement and indulge the fortuitous whims and luck of the stroller, there remain only superficial sights, cities that dwindle from view, buildings enhanced by alluring optical illusions. Not only am I determined, from now and henceforward, to remain satisfied with this state of affairs, but I am stimulated by the prospect.

Thinking of pain as a potential fuel for life-fulfilling activities is not as contradictory as it sounds when you realize that pain is, in fact, a form of energy.

Pain as Energy

As we saw in Chapter 2, both pain messages and our emotional reactions to them are actually biochemical impulses transmitted along the complex pathways of the brain and nervous system. You might think of pain as firing off a dizzying cycle of electrical activity along these paths. In acute pain these messages accomplish something: there is a great flurry of activity in the body, aimed at responding to a perceived physical emergency. In the case of an injury, for example, a veritable host of healing forces is summoned to the wound. But with chronic pain, our circuits are loaded with an unbelievable amount of information that has nowhere to go but around and around. Unless you intercept it. If all those messages could glow, a person with chronic pain could probably light up the Empire State Building. Imagine what you could do with all that energy if you could release it from the short circuit of chronic pain. You can start a bonfire by focusing the sun's rays through a simple lens. Giant mirrors now collect and harness solar energy for just about every use known to humankind. By training yourself to focus the energy of pain you can use it for almost any purpose you set your mind to.

Harnessing the Energy of Pain: The Wisdom of Aikido

One of the most ingenious ways of thinking about energy is the concept that provides the basis for the ancient Japanese martial art known as *aikido* — "the art of being centered." In *aikido* when you are attacked you do not counterattack; you simply take the force of your attacker and turn it back on him or her. You yourself, by not opposing force with force, remain centered and unhurt. In *The Ultimate Athlete*, George Leonard conveys an outsider's first astonished glimpse of this extraordinary art:

> The defender takes his stand on the mat. He is relaxed yet alert. He offers none of the exotic defensive poses popularized by the movie and television action thrillers. An attacker rushes at him, but he remains calm and still until the last instant. There follows a split second of unexpected intimacy in which the two figures, attacker and attacked, seem to merge. The attacker is sucked into a whirlpool of motion, then flung through the air *with little or no effort on the part of the defender,* who ends the maneuver in the same relaxed posture [italics mine].

The concept of an "aikido response" to pain may help you move toward freeing and using the energy supplied by chronic pain. According to *aikido,* a person's center is the *ki,* a kind of spiritual, mental, and physical center of gravity all rolled into one. If your *ki* is strong, no one can catch you off guard. The guiding principle is to use the most economical movement to accomplish your goal; a mere flick of the wrist can send an attacker sprawling on his back. The traditional movements of this nonaggressive, dancelike art flow into each other so organically that it is difficult to tell where attack leaves off and defense begins.

You can practice *aikido* in your mind without ever setting foot in a traditional Japanese practice space. The mental key is to think of *transformation and substitution at the same time,* so that you take the force of a specific time span of pain (an hour, a day) and immediately convert that energy into an equally energetic action or thought of your own choosing.

One man I interviewed had taught himself the rudiments of jewelry making from a book. When his pain was strong he found the greatest satisfaction in producing handsome rings made, of all things, from dimes. These he gave away to friends, enjoying once again the sense of having turned his pain into something tangible and beautiful.

Rosalie, whose pain is always worse after her day at work, comes home, takes a hot bath, and then, after a short nap, channels her pain energy into vivid surrealistic paintings. "It's funny," she told me, "but the worse the pain is, the more involved I get with my painting."

Bill, a disabled steelworker, told me he had started going to auctions every Saturday night to collect bits and pieces for his new hobby of making collages. "I go even when the pain is bad," he said, "but my wife won't go with me. She says it's all a lot of junk. I buy things that look like garbage to her. She doesn't understand that I'm looking past the dirt and grime to the object as it really is." Bill was *choosing* to see things differently. His eyes were open to the potential for transformation in objects other people had decided to scrap.

You can use the energy of pain to fuel your own transformations. It's up to you to figure out where your own interests and capabilities lie and how you want to use them. If nothing comes immediately to mind, glance back at the lists on page 108 and focus on one of the activities from List 2 or List 3. Whatever you choose, the point is to use your interests consciously to take the place of pain.

A diagram of the process might look something like this:

The arrow shows that the direction of energy is simultaneously in and out: the "attack" of pain is immediately turned outward (instead of being accepted or turned against yourself through resignation or depression or despair), as if you yourself had generated all the energy. This is the *aikido* response to pain.

The techniques that follow present a range of approaches for focusing the energy of pain and maximizing your ability to turn it around.

Framing

One of people's greatest fears when pain starts up is that it's going to get worse. On top of the pain they're feeling at the moment, they feel the pain they think or fear is just around the corner. The typical thought process goes something like this: "If it's this bad at four o'clock, imagine how awful it will be by six. *Then* what will I do?" When you're in pain and thinking ahead to more, you are projecting. Projection=Pitfall=Pain. Projection is an almost guaranteed method for perpetuating pain *ad infinitum*. The opposite of projection is *framing*. By framing your pain, instead of seeing yourself floating in an endless sea of pain, you visualize *non*-pain on both sides of a given episode.

Let's say it's Sunday morning and you wake up in pain. The immediate frame you construct begins with Saturday, which, just to make things easy, we'll say was relatively pain-free. Now, visualizing the free and easy space of Saturday, you proceed to build a time sandwich, with pain in the middle. Pick an outside frame that is realistic but optimistic; let your past experience be your guide. Even if you figure on a Sunday in pain, if you can visualize that one day framed between two days of *non*-pain, you're already in good shape.

By framing your pain when it first starts up, you give yourself the message that it's not going to last forever and keep getting worse. What framing also does is give you a way of focusing the energy of pain. If you expect pain all day Sunday, you can decide what you're going to do to keep it at a minimum (the ecology of pain) and how you're going to use and redirect its energy (*aikido* response).

Getting Rid of Residual Misery

> There is a Languor of the Life
> More imminent than Pain —
> 'Tis Pain's successor — When the Soul
> Has suffered all it can —
>
> EMILY DICKINSON

Framing also helps eliminate what I call "residual misery" — the feeling of sadness and immobility that lingers *after* pain. How often have you suddenly realized that you've been out of pain for several hours — and that instead of lying around you could actually have been up and about? Residual misery can be firmly and serenely nudged away if you visualize the outer frame of a given episode as a line you step across and leave behind you. Just imagine a crack in a sidewalk and you'll know exactly what I mean. Once you've crossed that line, residual misery is behind you.

Because everyone's pain is so different — and because even your own can have more than one pattern — you will need to adapt framing and the techniques that follow to fit your specific situation. If your pain is episodic, you can frame pain by painlessness or very low-grade pain; if your pain is more or less constant, framing can help you isolate the periods of intensest pain against a background of more manageable pain. Once you have framed a given episode of pain or part of an episode (you can frame five minutes if you want to), you are ready to turn its energy into life energy. Remember, the key is *substitution and transformation at the same time.* The turnaround of energy (ↄ) comes from being clear about your goals and not adding needless extra energy to that already supplied by pain.

Visualizing the Turnaround

Aikido masters use visualizations to help their disciples feel the energy of their *ki*. A typical suggestion is to think of a pulse just below your navel, from which a flow of energy radiates upward through your body, streaming into your arms, down into your hands, and out through your fingertips into the air, pouring back down toward the center of the earth like a waterfall. By concentrating on this sort of imagery, students of *aikido* develop a fluid strength without any evidence of muscular tension.

A similar mental image can help you make the turnaround

from pain energy into life energy. By establishing a one-to-one correlation between your pain and its substitute, you will be able to imagine a continuous flow between them. The more adept you become at visualizing this sort of transformation, the easier it will be for you to carry the practice into "real" life.

The first step is to be as precise as possible in defining exactly what you are going to do with the energy from your pain. Let's say you've framed an hour of pain. You might think aloud, for example, "My knees are throbbing and I'm going to ———" (read one chapter from the novel I started last month and never got back to), or "My back hurts and I'm going to ———" (answer that letter from So-and-So that's been lying on my desk), or "My headache hasn't subsided and I'm going to ———" (glue the Mexican ashtray the cat knocked off the kitchen table yesterday).

When you've got your pain and its equivalent clearly in focus, you're ready to begin. As you very slowly inhale, preferably with your eyes closed, imagine the flow of pain coming into your body through the soles of your feet, passing through the "afflicted parts," and going back out through your feet as life energy as you exhale it with a continuous motion into the activity of your choice. Again, be as specific as you can. Visualize every motion you will make in carrying out the activity you have chosen in place of pain. See yourself picking up the book, opening it, and using the energy of pain to read, understand, and appreciate the words on the page. Now open your eyes. The rehearsal is over and the show can begin.

A little pain energy can go a long way. If you're feeling pretty good, it can keep you going. If you're not quite ready to take on the world, it can help you make the phone call that will put you in touch with someone you'd enjoy talking with or who can give you the information you need about your library card renewal, adult education courses in your community, vocational rehabilitation programs, or a group you've been thinking of joining, just to suggest a few examples.

Remember, when you use it, that all that energy didn't come from you; it came from pain. There's no end to the ingenious uses you can make of it once you get started.

Tapping the Energy of Anger

Anger may be one of the most overlooked and potentially one of the most useful components of the chronic pain experience. To judge from the testimony of all the men and women I interviewed, it is one of the most common reactions to protracted pain. Did they actually say they were angry? Not in so many words until I asked them directly. Anger is rarely obvious. More often than not, it masquerades as resignation, acceptance, defiance, or despair. It would rather don the cloak of martyrdom or machismo than declare itself.

The main reason people are angry at pain is because it limits them. For some people the limits are slight, for some they are severe. Whatever your situation, if pain has limited your activities — whether by keeping you from taking part in a favorite sport, by preventing you from holding a full-time job or finishing your studies, or by making it impossible for you to shop alone or drive — repressing your anger can be even more crippling than the pain itself. When you repress it, anger turns against you by becoming a pain compounder. When you don't express it, it can suddenly explode against the very people you love most. But if you learn to deal with anger simply and openly, it can become a powerful tool for focusing your *aikido* response to pain. Why? Because anger itself is a kernel of smoldering energy.

The first step in learning to use anger is recognizing that

s there. When you've done everything you can to bring our pain down to at least a necessary level and you still have pain, a certain amount of anger is inevitable. How much depends on how limiting your pain is, and how you react to those particular limits.

Step two is digging it out from under its various disguises. We lose the power anger could supply by squirreling it away under a heap of secondary, deenergizing feelings. Naturally, none of us can live for long in a state of unrelieved fury. But *by spending a few self-aware minutes* focusing on our anger we can regain the power the pain compounders drain away.

Anger comes in all sizes. The key to using it is making it specific (echoes of framing). Being angry "at pain" is much too vague. When you know exactly what you're angry *at*, you can release the energy of pain, slingshot style, by substituting a positive situation for one of difficulty or impossibility.

Let's say your rheumatoid arthritis makes it pretty excruciating for you to dance. You're seeing someone new and dancing would be a nice activity to share. You still have a lot of choices. You can go dancing anyway (masochist). You can be sad and resigned and say with a sigh, "I wish I could . . ." (defeatist). You can feel sorry for yourself and probably elicit some pity from your friend (martyr). Or, before you disappear forever into the slough of despair, you can get in touch with your anger and use it to propel you toward a different activity that you and your new friend might equally, or almost equally, enjoy.

The conversation in your head goes as follows:

> I'm angry!
> (Angry at what?)
> Angry at my pain.
> (Be more specific.)
> At the pain in my legs!
> (Why are you angry at the pain in your legs?)

Because it keeps me from dancing!
(When?)
While my arthritis is bad.
(How long has that been?)
For two months.
(Why are you angry right now?)
Because I want to go dancing tomorrow night.
(Why are you thinking about that now?)
Because I have to make plans with X!

Now you've got it really narrowed down in time and space. You're not angry forever. You're angry right now. Instead of getting chronically depressed or defeated, you can take the energy of this specific anger and use it to deal with a specific, relatively small, but nonetheless sobering limitation on your new relationship. What can you do instead of going dancing? That's up to you.

The wisdom of *aikido* will help you visualize a graphic turnaround of negative energy into something positive you yourself have made happen. Your anger at what you *can't* do is the flick of the wrist that makes the arrow of pain spin back toward what you *can* do.

The same techniques can be applied to all sorts of moments in the day when chronic pain interferes with what you want to do or have to do.

Jack's gout was so painful that he was having trouble concentrating on all the marketing reports he had to read and analyze at work. Jack didn't say he was angry until I asked him directly. What he expressed first was depression and fear — fear that he'd fall further and further behind until he lost his job. He was also frightened because his soldierly determination to win out over the pain wasn't working. If Jack had been more aware of his anger and had known how to use it, his ability to concentrate would have dramatically improved. His inner dialogue might sound like this:

> I'm frightened.
> (Are you sure you aren't angry? Pain compounders should always arouse a suspicion of anger lurking underneath.)
> Yes, I'm angry!
> (Angry at what?)
> Angry at my pain.
> (Be more specific.)
> At the pain in my hands!
> (Why are you angry at the pain in your hands?)
> Because it's keeping me from doing my work.
> (Why? Does it keep you from writing?)
> No, it keeps me from concentrating!
> (Why?)
> Because I don't know what's causing it. I'm afraid it's a symptom of something fatal.
> (When does it keep you from concentrating?)
> Every day.
> (Keep narrowing it down. Is it keeping you from concentrating right now?)
> Yes!
> (How long has that been going on?)
> Ten minutes.
> (Can you stop now and do something about it?)
> Yes!

With ten minutes' worth of anger — and the realization that a great deal of his pain is being compounded by worry — Jack's best bet would be to spend ten minutes on the phone making an appointment with his doctor. Jack needs to know what is causing his pain. Once he puts his fears to rest, his hand pain will probably cause him less distress. If he is able to keep up with his work load, he won't be angry at his pain — at least not for *that* reason.

Sometimes pain produces angers that loom larger than these. If your pain is associated with a permanent or protracted disability, particularly if it relates to an aspect of your life that is especially meaningful, you will be faced with an anger that has no obvious or easy equivalent. If you are a ballet dancer with severe arthritis or a carpenter with crippled hands, your grief (and consequent anger) will probably be far greater than that of the person who has trouble climbing stairs or whose hands no longer have the strength to open jars.

One woman, a hairdresser who could no longer stand because of injuries she had sustained in a terrible accident, was slowly beginning to reassess her options:

> "It's hard. Hard even to know what I want to do. No matter what your profession is — a doctor, a lawyer, a beautician, a psychologist — you become good at what you do. Then all of a sudden you have to change everything."

If the lifework you had set out for yourself is no longer feasible, it may take months of careful planning, perhaps with the help of an expert career counselor, before you can reassess your abilities and begin to reorient yourself in a new direction.*

One man I interviewed spoke of using his anger in ways he would feel proud of, instead of turning it against himself. His chronic back pain fueled his work as a writer, perhaps all the more so because he had had to give up a promising career as an athlete.

There can also be a more generalized anger, if pain is part

* See the Coping Resource Guide beginning on page 231 for suggestions about counseling and vocational retraining.

of a condition that disfigures or disables you in ways that make you feel less capable or less attractive or just plain "sidelined." Chronic pain, when linked to a major loss — whether of livelihood, vocation, or sense of sexual well-being — can be a constant reminder of that loss.

Paul's back operation left scars that went below the surface:

> "I've lost confidence in my body as a vehicle to do for me what I need. It's not something I can count on, it's unreliable — I mean, it broke down, it gave out. It let me down. I used to believe that I could do whatever I needed to do to make things right ... Now, I don't have the capability to insure that. But it's not just physical things, it's — well, everything. I'm doing less, I'm less able to cope."

When Jack's gout intensified, the weakness in his hands was a blow to his whole self-image:

> "My hands used to be the strongest part of my body. I could kill with my hands. Now they're reduced to things dropping from them. I'm afraid sometimes that I could drop my grandchild. Before, my hands were something I could open things with. I could do almost anything with them. Now I have nothing."

Learning to cope with this sort of pain involves confronting the rage beneath the surface. Anger of this dimension *can* be turned around, but in order to do full justice to your needs and aspirations, as well as the depth of your feeling, you may have to use it in a larger, more long-range way.

Anger can fuel your job-hunting efforts, as well as your return to school for further study or specialized training. It can also spur your involvement with social or political groups that are working to improve health care delivery in ways that might benefit you or others with a condition similar to yours. Long-term commitments, whether to new interests, new work, new people, or an active role in your community, are an *aikido* response writ large.

Anger at chronic pain is not a feeling you deal with once and then leave blissfully behind. So long as your pain persists or recurs, anger will be there wagging its tail. You will be dealing with your pain most healthily when you make dealing with anger a conscious tool in your pain repertoire. Anger can undermine you terribly if you lose it to the pain compounders. But it can be a powerful ally in your struggle to live with chronic pain if you learn to use it.

■ ■ ■

Once you have gotten a sense of your pain as a concentrated form of energy — through such techniques as framing, visualizing the turnaround, and tapping the energy of anger — you should begin to feel like the possessor of a powerful new tool. It may take a while before you fully assimilate the idea of an *aikido* response to pain and actually put it to work in your own life. For the moment, however, the important thing to keep in mind is the essence: don't contribute to the struggle, use it. How you use the struggle of pain will depend on your particular goals, temperament, and interests, which the next chapter will help you explore. When you are in touch with where you're going, you won't be thrown by the energy of pain. Like a skilled practitioner of *aikido*, you will simply take its thrust and redirect it — wherever you choose.

PART III

The
Follow-Through

8

Setting New Goals

The difficult I'll do right now; the impossible takes a little time.

BILLIE HOLIDAY

"Most people," writes Dr. Frederic F. Flach in his book *Choices*, "can look back over the years and identify a time and place at which their lives changed significantly. Whether by accident or design, these are the moments when, because of a readiness within us and a collaboration with events occurring around us, we are forced to seriously reappraise ourselves and the conditions under which we live and to make certain choices that will affect the rest of our lives."

Having read this far, you are probably at such a point yourself. Moments of reappraisal are turning points — rare, exciting pauses that signal a beginning of sorts, a new chapter in our lives. Of course, chronic pain in and of itself does not exactly generate excitement; but when you have glimpsed the light at the end of the tunnel and begun to turn your pain energy around and *use* it, you have ample cause for rejoicing.

The pages that follow are actually a model planning session disguised as a chapter in a book. They are a place to catch your breath, take stock of where you are with your pain, and figure out where you go from here.

Identity Crisis

I remember sitting in a doctor's waiting room about a year after I first got sick. While I was leafing through a magazine, the next patient, a man in his middle forties, arrived. As he was taking off his coat I heard the receptionist say, "You're a lower back?" "No, upper," the man replied.

Both the receptionist and the patient were unconsciously perpetuating one of the most disabling aspects of the chronic pain experience: the labels that equate the person with the pain. You are *not* your pain. Overwhelming as your pain may often be, it is only one part of your whole life. One of the most important stages in learning to live with chronic pain is putting your pain in its place, which means putting it in perspective.

Putting Your Pain in Perspective

You are infinitely larger than your pain. Because many factors besides pain make you the person you are today, your life surrounds and encompasses your pain. Sometimes just being able to visualize the sweep of important events and experiences that compose the time line of your life can give you a sense of where your pain fits into the full spectrum of your life.

The following exercise is adapted from a technique introduced by Tristine Rainer in her book *The New Diary*.

Think back on your life. Beginning with your own birth, list the most significant events or experiences — both positive and negative — of your life so far. Include the important turning points in your personal, work, and career experience. Indicate by closest approximate date the onset of your pain, but do *not* include any other health-related episodes unless they specifically affect or have affected your pain.

Sample Entry	Your Entry
I was born on November 10, 1934.	I was born on
1. 1938: "Baby" sister born	1.
2. 1939: Started school	2.
3. 1942: Father killed in action	3.
4. 1950: Decided to be a singer	4.
5. 1952: Scholarship to conservatory	5.
6. 1955: Marriage to Jim	6.
7. 1956: First daughter born	7.
8. 1956: The car crash. Pain begins	8.
9. 1959: Second daughter born	9.

Sample Entry	Your Entry
10. 1965: Started singing again	10.
11. 1969: Split with Jim	11.
12. 1969: M.A. in counseling	12.
13. 1971: Operation on my bad leg	13.
14. 1974: Cathy off to college	14.
15. 1975: New job and new lover	15.
16. 1977: Anne off; I'm on my own	16.

How long have you been in chronic pain, and what fraction of your lifetime do those months or years represent? Most important of all, what *else* has happened in your life since pain began? If your list of key experiences stops where pain starts, it's time for you to get back on the track of your life. The rest of this chapter will help you plan a coping strategy so you can do just that, based on your own assessment of your strengths and weaknesses and your short- and long-term goals.

Setting New Goals

By setting pain-coping goals for the long term (six months or more) and the more immediate future (the next four weeks), you aren't signing your life away to chronic pain. If your condition is self-limiting, or heals, or simply vanishes, what could be better? By setting forth your goals all you are doing is stating your commitment to handling your pain in the best way you know how *if* you still have it in the months to come. More than anything else, this is a message to yourself, your way of saying, "It matters. I matter. I *can* be in less pain and I will. I'm on the path to pain control."

Sticking It Out on the Island

You may recall the story of Robinson Crusoe, who spent twenty-eight years shipwrecked on an island and survived — in the person of Daniel Defoe — to tell his extraordinary tale. After he had notched off a year's worth of lines on his improvised calendar, Crusoe sat down, in his words, "to consider seriously my condition."

> I drew up the state of my affairs in writing not so much to leave them to any that were to come after me (for I was like to have but few heirs), as to deliver my thoughts from daily poring upon them, and afflicting my mind; and I stated very impartially, like debtor and creditor, the comforts I enjoyed against the miseries I suffered, thus:

Evil	Good
I am cast upon a horrible desolate island, void of all hope of recovery.	But I am alive; and not drowned, as all my ship's company were.
I have no clothes to cover me . . .	But I am in a hot climate, where if I had clothes, I could hardly wear them . . .

When Crusoe had finished, he concluded that there was no condition so wretched but that "we may always find in it something to comfort ourselves from, and to set . . . on the credit side of the account."

Being stranded in the land of pain can be just as lonely and desperate as being shipwrecked off the coast of South America. Yet in pain too there may be credits to be set against the negative side of the ledger. As you prepare to spell out your long- and short-term goals for coping, it is a good idea to be aware of just what those credits are for you. In the space provided below or separately in your Pain Journal make your own list of "good" and "evil," following Robinson Crusoe's lead and the sample given.

Evil	Good
My body hurts (be specific — where?).	Being in pain has made me more aware of my body and value it more.
I can't take part in sports.	I've started playing the guitar again after all these years.
It's hard for me to take public transportation and I can't afford taxis.	I go out less but I'm planning more social events in my house.
I have trouble sleeping.	I've done a lot of crossword puzzles and read a lot of novels.
I can't be as politically active as I used to be.	I write a lot of letters to the editor and I've gotten involved in the health care movement.

And now it's your turn:

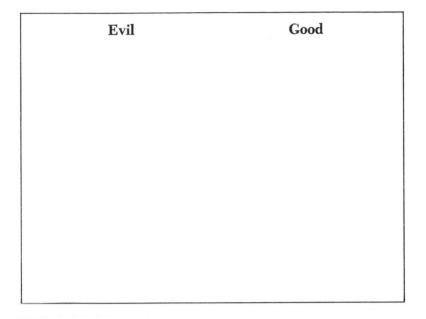

Evil	Good

Primary Gains

Health professionals use the phrase "secondary gain" to refer to an illness-related gain, whether financial (economic compensation) or personal (extra attention), that interferes with a person's ability to return to a productive life following an injury or illness. If a secondary gain is involved, chronic pain or any other long-term medical problem can become a self-perpetuating excuse for staying out of work, not taking responsibility for your half of a mature relationship, or failing to develop your talents in any other way.

Instances of secondary gain certainly exist; we all have to fight them. But how many health professionals, ever vigilant for cases of secondary gain, take the time to focus on the *primary* gain a person may experience as a result of injury or illness?

A primary gain is one which is yours to keep *whether or not your illness persists*. Not everyone experiences a primary gain, but in many cases being ill or in pain can change your awareness of yourself so that even when and if you recover you will carry your changed perception with you. Pain, when you learn to listen to its message, can be a catalyst or teacher, acting as a force for change that sends you back to old interests or hobbies or takes you in new directions that might not otherwise have opened up to you.

For example, you may, like Colette, find unexpected joys in the slower rhythms and adaptations dictated by illness. When her arthritis had become so severe that she could no longer walk, she wrote with gusto of her excursions by wheelchair:

> On my outings I drive along at the leisurely pace of a lady of the Second Empire. A pony-chaise could overtake me. There is always so much to look at when one travels slowly. Contrasting beauties effaced by speed fall into their proper perspective. My years and infirmities have surely earned me the right to go slow, to stop at whim beside a narcissus, a purple orchis, or a wild strawberry! . . . In the long run there is something to be said for having arthritis.

I could list a number of primary gains from my own experience of pain. First on the list would have to be my return to playing the cello, which has probably provided a richer source of happiness — and taken me further toward a more painless state of being — than any other "therapy" I've tried since I became sick. I had played seriously before I entered college, but only intermittently after that. Almost by instinct, partly because I was afraid the pain and weakness would spread to my arms, I gravitated back toward the cello within weeks of the first symptoms. Since then it has become a major activity; I've returned to studying and have begun to play chamber music. At this point I have trouble carrying such a large instrument, but I've had the great good luck to live in a neighborhood full of musicians, with playing possibilities in my own building as well as in a two-block radius. In addition, being in pain and having to lead a restricted life has opened my eyes to what it might feel like to be old. My own feeling was echoed by Rosalie, who hopes one day to start a self-sufficient crafts community where old people would train young apprentices in arts and trades that are gradually being lost.

I've become keenly aware, too, in a way I never would have otherwise, of the terrible inequities in our current health care system. I experienced at first hand what it is like to go undiagnosed for so long. I experienced condescending treatment from male doctors that utterly shocked me. I experienced malpractice — of a minor sort. I had three muscle biopsies, relatively trivial but nonetheless invasive, painful, and scarring procedures. One was incompletely written up and thus was useless to subsequent physicians who examined me. The second was dropped in a solution that made it impossible to carry out all the tests the doctor had ordered. The third, performed to put matters right once and for all, was lost in the mail between Boston and New York. I came away from all these experiences changed and angry, particularly when I realized that my own experience was tame compared to that of many others. As a middle-class person I had received what is known as "thorough workups" from the "best" hospitals. I have since, to end the story happily, found a superb physician. Still, I know how much work we will all have to do before we have a health system in this country that respects all its patients and all its personnel.

Many of the people I interviewed mentioned one or more primary gains. This brings us full circle from the inherited interpretations that were discussed in Chapter 3. Your pain may not have made you more virtuous or "deeper" than you were before, but it may have brought you a primary gain that you can state in your own terms. If so, you may want to use the space provided below or your Pain Journal to record for yourself what you feel you have gained from pain.

Primary Gains

We're almost ready. Before turning to the self-help charts on pages 143–46, you may want to flip back to the questions you asked yourself on page 48. How many of those have now been answered? How many are still pending? You might also take a peek at the action chart on page 62, as well as at the list of possibilities you filled in on page 108. Have you put any of these plans and possibilities in motion?

One last point. In setting goals for any project it is always a good idea to include at least two or three objectives you can be sure of attaining. This gives you a built-in, guaranteed sense of satisfaction to balance out the more challenging aspects of your plans. If all your goals are difficult, you're planting the seeds of guaranteed failure. You want to challenge yourself, but not to the point of folly. An example of a highly attainable "insti-goal" might be:

■ I'm going to replace the burnt-out light bulb in the lamp on my night table so I'll be able to read in bed without craning my neck and having to get up to turn out the overhead light.

Taking Stock: A Bird's-Eye View of Your Coping Abilities

Without giving it a lot of thought, simply list what you consider your strongest qualities for coping — those personality traits and attitudes that could or do give you a generous push along the path to pain control:

1.

2.

3.

Today's Date _____ **My Pain Level Right Now** _____
(see page 34)

The next time I'm in pain,

instead of _____
(a response you know only makes things worse)

I'm going to try _____
(a response you think has a chance of helping)

Long-Term Goals

If I still have pain six months from now, I'd like to be able to look back at this page and have made the changes listed under **Goals:**

Goals	How I'll Proceed
1. Fill in these areas of medical ignorance:	Steps I can take to learn about each:
a.	a.
b.	b.
c.	c.
2. Eliminate these three physical factors that increase my pain:	I'll do this by (give approach for each):
a.	a.
b.	b.
c.	c.
3. Deal with the following pain compounders:	I'll begin work on each of them by:
a.	a.
b.	b.
c.	c.
4. Try these new hobbies or activities (include at least one that involves you with other people):	First step toward each of these:
a.	a.
b.	b.
c.	c.

5. Make these changes in my living arrangements, both physical and social:

I'll get started on each one by:

a.

a.

b.

b.

c.

c.

6. Maximize these areas of personal strength:

How I can bring out these aspects of my character:

a.

a.

b.

b.

c.

c.

7. Minimize these aspects of my response to pain:

How I can reduce each of these:

a.

a.

b.

b.

c.

c.

Work

8. Specific goals relating to employment:

First step I need to take for each:

a.

a.

b.

b.

c.

c.

Outreach

9. Groups or specific people I'd like to reach out to:

First step I need to take to get involved with each:

a.

a.

b.

b.

c.

c.

Self-Portrait: Future Tense

If I still have pain six months from now, this is how I'd like to see myself:

Short-Term Goals

In the next four weeks I'm going to take the following steps toward setting my Long-Term Goals in motion: (Look back at your Long-Term Goals. Short-Term Goals come straight from "How I'll Proceed." For numbers 1 through 9, simply list step a, and you'll be well on your way!)

1.
2.
3.
4.
5.
6.
7.
8.
9.

Use this space for two "insti-goals" you can be absolutely sure of attaining:

1.
2.

9

To Take or Not to Take: The Pros and Cons of the Most Widely Prescribed Painkillers

Is it time for my painkiller?

HAM, in Samuel Beckett's
Endgame

The human species is distinguished from the lower
orders by its desire to take medicine.

SIR WILLIAM OSLER

You may be wondering why a chapter on drugs, which after
all are such a central part of the chronic pain experience,
appears so far along in a book on pain control. The answer
is simple. Drugs can be an extraordinary help in coping
with pain, but they need to be seen in the broadest possible
context. Drugs are only one tool among the many you now
possess.

The issue of drugs is an emotional one, and it is one on
which people are quick to take sides or jump to extreme

positions. Painkillers for chronic pain — absolutely not, many doctors will tell you; if aspirin doesn't do it, try gritting your teeth. Chronic pain — relieve it by all means, the drug companies proclaim through multimillion-dollar advertising campaigns. With the horrific rise in drug addiction we have seen in recent years, a cloud of fear and misinformation has gathered around the use of all drugs. As a result, people with chronic pain have no clear source of information on the very drugs we are most likely to receive from doctors — painkillers.

You have the right to your own attitude toward painkillers. You also have the right to base your opinions on solid, scientific information. This chapter has been designed as a reference section that will guide you swiftly and succinctly through the jargon of pharmacology to what you really need to know about the painkillers you are now using or may eventually consume.* In the pages that follow we will take a look at the uses and misuses of the seven primary painkillers listed below. We'll focus on what you need to know before you use them; how you can use them for maximum effectiveness; and how they may interact with the other medications listed, as well as with alcohol.

The Seven Primary Painkillers**

- aspirin and aspirin compounds
- Tylenol (acetaminophen)
- codeine and codeine compounds

* For a fuller guide to the wise use of *all* medication, see *The People's Pharmacy* by Joe Graedon or its excellent companion volume, *The People's Pharmacy 2* by Joe Graedon and Teresa Graedon. A more detailed work, also highly recommended, is *The Doctors' and Patients' Handbook of Medicines and Drugs* by Peter Parish.
** The most common brand name is given first, with generic name in parentheses. Where the generic name is better known, drugs are named without brand.

- Darvon (propoxyphene) and Darvon compounds
- Percodan (oxycodone, aspirin, phenacetin, and caffeine) and Percocet (oxycodone and acetaminophen)
- Talwin (pentazocine) and Talwin compound
- Demerol (meperidine)

Drugs you may also be taking for treatment of your pain or the underlying medical condition that produces your pain are:

ANTI-INFLAMMATORIES
Butazolidin (phenylbutazone)
Clinoril (sulindac)
Indocin (indomethacin)
Motrin (ibuprofen)
Naprosyn (naproxen)

MUSCLE RELAXANTS
Robaxin (methocarbamol)
Soma (carisoprodol)
Valium (diazepam)

STEROIDS
cortisone
prednisone

DRUGS FOR GOUT
Colchicine
and anti-inflammatories

DRUGS FOR MIGRAINE
ergotamine
Inderal (propranolol)
Sansert (methysergide)

DRUGS FOR ANGINA
Inderal (propranolol)
nitroglycerin

Other drugs doctors often prescribe for people with chronic pain include:

TRANQUILIZERS AND ANTIDEPRESSANTS
Valium (diazepam)
Librium (chlordiazepoxide)
Miltown (meprobamate)
Elavil (amitriptyline)
Sinequan (doxepin)
Tofranil (imipramine)

SLEEPING PILLS
Dalmane (flurazepam)
Nembutal (pentobarbital)
Seconal (secobarbital sodium)

Some Basic Definitions

I know of no clearer working definition of the word *drug* than the one given by Dr. Peter Parish:

> A drug may be defined as any substance which can alter the structure or function of the living organism. Air pollutants, pesticides, vitamins, and virtually any chemical may be regarded as drugs. Therefore, all medicines are drugs, but not all drugs are medicines. Those drugs used as medicines have been selected because they possess or are thought to possess useful properties.

Because of confusion about what drugs really are, and because of the widespread publicity about addiction and fatal drug overdose, many people with chronic pain are afraid to take any painkiller but aspirin. Ada Rogers, clinical coordinator of the Analgesic Studies Section at Memorial Sloan-Kettering Institute for Cancer Research, believes that many patients may suffer needlessly because of confusion regarding what constitutes "addiction."

Addiction: The word *addiction* has become so highly charged that many health professionals have begun to replace it with the term "drug dependence."

Drug Dependence: A condition in which the user has a compulsive desire to continue taking a drug either because of its "positive" (mood-enhancing) effects or in order to avoid the unpleasant effects that might result from its absence.

There are two kinds of drug dependence, psychological and physical. They can exist separately or together. Repeated administration of a drug can result in a physical condition in which the body craves the drug. Abrupt cessation of the drug can produce withdrawal symptoms if a person is physically dependent. However, in the absence of psychological dependence, physical dependence is not necessarily a hazardous condition. For example, you may become physically dependent on morphine following an operation for back surgery, but once the pain has begun to ebb and the drug is gradually withdrawn, you do not return home "addicted." Gradual withdrawal is essential to avoid unpleasant and sometimes dangerous symptoms that can occur with abrupt cessation.

Conversely, you can become psychologically dependent on a drug without physical dependence. For example, you may consistently take a certain medicine — say, codeine — because it makes you feel good instead of for its medicinal purpose, the relief of pain. Psychological dependence *in combination with* physical dependence is what most people really fear. Statistically, this is a rare combination indeed when analgesics are taken for medicinal purposes. By learning to use drugs with reasonable caution — in the right doses for you, under the right conditions for absorption, and for their correct medical purposes — you should be able to seek pain relief without fear of "addiction." According to Dr. Parish:

> On the whole, dependence seems most likely to arise when *three factors come together:* a potential drug of dependence, a "vulnerable" personality, and some adverse aspect of the environment. Whether the risk becomes reality depends on many other complex sociopsychological factors affecting that particular individual [italics mine].

Drug Tolerance: If certain drugs are taken repeatedly over time, higher doses may be required to produce the same effect. Most of us don't think of alcohol as a drug, so you may not have noticed when the glass of scotch that set you on your ear as a teenager became a pleasant drink. With certain painkillers, tolerance can be a problem for three reasons. It can make pain management difficult because of the need for constant readjustment of doses. Higher doses sometimes trigger disagreeable side effects such as drowsiness, nausea, or constipation. Finally, as you become tolerant to a drug, you take higher and higher doses to obtain the same effect. With certain premixed combinations you will also be getting higher and higher doses of other ingredients, such as aspirin, acetaminophen, or caffeine, which your body may not be able to handle. Tolerance can be reversed. It can also be avoided by the judicious use of the drugs you take. Before moving on to practical suggestions for the best use of pain medication, let's summarize what's been said so far with a simple lineup of facts and misconceptions.

MISCONCEPTION	FACT
Painkillers are addictive.	In most cases, "addiction" resides less in the drug itself than in a combination of personal, physiological, and environmental factors.
People with chronic pain are prime candidates for addiction: "Once you start, you'll never stop."	Unless you have reason to believe that you have what psychologists have called an "addictive personality" (a history of alcoholism might be a sign to watch for), there is no reason to fear that you will become dependent on painkillers if you use them properly.
The more you take painkillers, the less they will help you.	Tolerance to some painkillers can develop with protracted use. But you can minimize this possibility by using drugs strategically.

Painkillers: What You Need to Know and Why

Drugs are not inherently good or bad. Penicillin is no more and no less benign a drug than codeine, which is commonly prescribed for moderate to severe pain. Both drugs are effective when used for the right purpose, both can cause serious side effects, and both can be used with confidence by a well-informed consumer.

Painkillers are a valuable part of the pharmacopoeia of Western medicine (and that of most other cultures as well). I, for one, am glad they exist. As with all other drugs, there is a responsible, scientific way to use them so that you get the maximum benefit with a minimum of side effects. My own practice is to use them carefully, rather sparingly, and only when I feel that a painkiller will make a decisive difference in my ability to function or will ease me out of severe discomfort. I also believe that every medical consumer should know the following basic facts about any drug he or she takes:

1. Name of drug and expected benefit
2. Approximate time lapse before drug takes effect
3. Approximate duration of action
4. Possible negative side effects, both short and long term
5. Potential interactions with:

    ■ other drugs, particularly tranquilizers and sleeping pills
    ■ alcohol
    ■ certain food substances

Ordinarily, this is the kind of information most doctors do not spontaneously share with patients. As a result, you may be taking four or five medications without the slightest idea of what they are supposed to do and what their individual and combined long-term effects may be on your system. When a physician's enigmatic scrawl isn't followed up by a clear overview on how to use a medication, *you* have to follow up with questions. Unfortunately, most people know so little about medicine that they aren't even sure what questions to ask doctors about the drugs they receive. Now you do know what to ask: you can refer to the five-point list above. This isn't just a plug for self-assertion in the doctor's office. Your own health is at stake. According to pharmacologist Joe Graedon, investigations have shown that anywhere from 50 to 80 percent of patients take their drugs at the wrong times, in the wrong dose (underdosing as well as overdosing can have serious consequences), or for the wrong purpose.*

If your doctor gives you a runaround on medication, you might want to quote the following portion of a speech given by the head of the Food and Drug Administration (FDA), Dr. Jere Edwin Goyan, at the National Press Club in November 1979: "I believe that people should, indeed must, actively participate in making decisions about their own health care, including the selection of prescription drugs. I would not want to swallow a pill about which I knew nothing, and I would not expect anyone else to do so either."

---

* Elderly patients would appear to be at special risk for errors in the use of medication. According to Graedon, a 1979 study conducted by Dr. Peter Lamy found drug prescribing for the elderly to be "extraordinarily high . . . It has been reported that more than 85 percent of elderly ambulatory patients and almost 95 percent of elderly institutionalized patients receive drugs, 25 percent of which may well be ineffective or unneeded." These figures are appalling when viewed along with the results of a 1978 survey of drug use among senior citizens in Albany, New York, which found that 83 percent were regularly using seven to fifteen drugs, and only 8 percent were completely medication-free, while 33 percent took one or more medications they could not specifically name. A survey of older people in Miami, Florida, produced similar statistics.

A special booklet, *Using Your Medicines Wisely: A Guide for the Elderly,* prepared by the National Institute on Drug Abuse, is available free of cost from Elder-Ed, P.O. Box 416, Kensington, MD. 20795.

How Painkillers Work

All painkillers are essentially symptomatic treatment, in that they treat the pain itself rather than its underlying cause. The term *analgesic* is used to refer to any drug that provides relief from pain. For our purposes, two very broad categories can be distinguished: "simple" analgesics and narcotic analgesics. It is very important to understand the difference between them.

Simple analgesics, of which aspirin is the prototype, combat pain at the site of injury or inflammation. Their exact mechanism of action is still poorly understood, but it is known that they inhibit the production of prostaglandins, which are pain mediators. Aspirin and aspirin compounds, as well as acetaminophen (Tylenol), are simple analgesics.

Narcotic analgesics, of which morphine is the prototype, owe their action to medicinal substances derived from the plant that produces opium. (These drugs are also referred to as "opiates.") Codeine, Darvon, Percodan, Talwin, and Demerol all belong in this category. These drugs differ from each other in chemical structure but are quite similar in action and effect. The narcotic analgesics do not act at the site of pain; they act on the central nervous system (brain and spinal cord) to alter our *perception* of pain. The pain itself remains, but the significance we attach to it is changed. All narcotic analgesics can cause tolerance, and all have the potential for abuse.

In using analgesics of either type, it is important to keep in mind that individual patients differ enormously in their reactions to medication.

The Facts on Side Effects

All drugs have side effects. Aspirin, the wonder drug, can cause irritation or ulceration in the lining of the stomach if you use it indiscriminately or are highly susceptible to it. Penicillin, another wonder drug, can cause death in those who are allergic to it. Most people do not experience drug reactions of such dire proportions. Nonetheless, there are striking differences in the way people absorb, metabolize, and eliminate particular drugs.

Before a painkiller can bring about its desired effect, it has to enter your body, either through the mouth (orally), fat or muscle (by injection), the bloodstream (intravenously), or the rectum (via suppositories, uncommon in the United States). Once a drug is absorbed, its overall effect is essentially *systemic*. This means that while it is taking effect in one part of your body, it may be producing the same effect three inches away, where you don't need any help at all. It may also set in motion an entirely different and unexpected process, such as building up fat between your shoulder blades when you thought it was supposed to be unfreezing your arthritic hip (cortisone may do this over time). Most drugs can't be aimed. Even injections into a specific painful part of the body are absorbed into the blood and have a system-wide effect. "No greater fallacy exists," Norman Cousins writes, . . . than that a drug is like an arrow that can be shot at a particular target. Its actual effect is more like a shower of porcupine quills."

It is up to you to be aware of how you are reacting to a given drug. Some people are more susceptible than others to certain side effects — gastric upset, for example, in reaction to aspirin or codeine. You may "process" a drug differently from one day to another, or from one period to another. As you age, your whole rate of metabolism slows, which means that drug doses need to be adjusted for age. Older people get appreciably longer action but also increased side effects from almost all medications.

You are the best judge of how a drug is affecting you. In using any medication, painkillers included, it is essential to weigh the benefits against any real or potential risks. If a drug is causing you nausea or giving you heartburn or making you overly dizzy, don't just chalk it up to side effects. Tell your doctor right away. There is probably another drug that can help you just as well without causing you distress.

When Should I Take Painkillers and Which Ones Should I Take?

These are tough questions to answer. If your pain is severe enough to interfere significantly with your ability to function and your sense of well-being, you might take Ham's question on page 147 and turn it into a statement: "It's time for my painkiller." On the other hand, all narcotic analgesics may cloud your perception and make it even *harder* for you to function. Narcotic analgesics like codeine and Darvon also make some people sleepy. If you are planning to drive a car or operate machinery of any kind (except perhaps a typewriter), you should think twice about taking a drug that is going to alter your perception of the road or slow your reflexes. However, if your pain is really bad, you probably won't be driving or operating power tools.

The guiding principle of pharmacology here is always to take the lowest dose of the weakest drug that will effectively relieve your pain. You don't start with sledgehammers like Talwin or Demerol. You start with aspirin or Tylenol. If they don't work, you and your doctor figure out which of the middle-range opiates might be more appropriate. Many physicians consider codeine with either aspirin or Tylenol a safe and highly effective combination, but that is only one possibility among many.

One recommendation: because of the risk of tolerance with narcotic analgesics, you will get the best long-term use out of drugs like codeine and Darvon by using them intermittently or in smaller combined doses, and only when you really need them. I've found it extremely helpful over the years to keep the Plain Ordinary Pain Scale (page 34) in mind before taking any drug for pain relief. Way back I made a sort of pact with myself: that only a level 6 pain rated medication. Over the years I've played a lot of games with those numbers, revising the scale so that what I used to call a level 6 is now a level 4. I credit this device with keeping me from developing tolerance, which means that I can still get substantial mileage out of the available drugs.

Aspirin

Aspirin, first synthesized for mass production in 1893, owes its wondrous powers to the willow tree, whose medicinal properties were recognized over two thousand years ago by the ancient Greeks and Romans. The Greeks chewed willow bark to ease the pains of childbirth; the Romans used it for sciatica. In this country, Native Americans were using willow tea as a cure for fever long before the European colonists arrived.

Today, twenty tons of aspirin are produced every day in the United States alone. Aspirin and aspirin-based compounds are used for a wide range of everyday complaints, from headaches to toothaches to the common cold, as well as in the treatment of many serious chronic illnesses. Because of its combined analgesic and anti-inflammatory action, aspirin is considered the drug of choice for most forms of arthritis. One of aspirin's strong points is that tolerance does not develop even when it's taken in large doses over many years. It is thus a highly effective drug for use in treating chronic pain.*

How to Take Aspirin

Aspirin should not be taken on an empty stomach. Some people find it is best mashed or dissolved in milk or water and taken with a small amount of food to minimize gastric upset. (A full meal can interfere with maximum absorption.) Some doctors recommend dissolving aspirin in a glass of seltzer or club soda, in the belief that the effervescent action facilitates absorption.

If gastric sensitivity develops even when you've taken all the foregoing precautions, it makes sense to try a buffered aspirin such as Arthritis Pain Formula, Ascriptin, or Bufferin. An enteric coated aspirin (Ecotrin) may be less well absorbed than either regular or buffered aspirin, so you're better off if you can take aspirin straight. Alcohol aggravates any gastrointestinal side effects of aspirin. A common side effect of too much aspirin is the sound of ringing in the ears.

Is There an Anacin Difference?

According to the physicians to whom I posed the question, no aspirin-type over-the-counter (OTC) medication is any more effective for pain than aspirin itself. (There may be good reasons for taking a different analgesic, but "extra" pain relief is not one of them.) Aspirin either works or it doesn't. The Anacin difference is basically no more than a clever advertising slogan; if you read the label closely, all it consists of is caffeine and an extra 75 mg. of aspirin above the usual 325 mg. contained in a single aspirin tablet. That's

---

* Aspirin can interfere with the retention of vitamin C in the body. If you are taking very high doses of aspirin, you should probably take supplementary vitamin C. Check with your physician.

the equivalent of adding a quarter-tablet more of aspirin and less than one cup of coffee!

For a detailed review of the many aspirin compounds now available in your local drugstore, once again see the invaluable *People's Pharmacy*.

Tylenol

Tylenol is *not* an aspirin product. It is an entirely different drug and, in certain cases, has distinct advantages over aspirin. For anyone who is sensitive or allergic to aspirin, Tylenol can be a useful substitute. (Anyone with stomach ulcers or blood-clotting problems should take Tylenol, not aspirin.) It is a simple analgesic that is effective for mild to moderate pain. However, Tylenol does not share aspirin's anti-inflammatory properties. Therefore, if your pain stems from a rheumatic or arthritic condition, Tylenol will not provide the same relief as aspirin.

Darvon

Darvon, a synthetic morphine-like agent that was first developed in the late 1960s, can be an effective middle-range painkiller for chronic pain of many different etiologies (origins). Nonetheless, some questions have been raised as to whether it is really as effective as initial studies seemed to promise. In addition, it can be habit forming. A number of reports now suggest that Darvon (along with Darvon Compound — propoxyphene and aspirin — and Darvocet — propoxyphene and acetaminophen) is actually more of a sedative than an analgesic.

The most frequently prescribed painkiller after aspirin, Darvon accounted for nearly 25 million retail prescriptions in 1980, which doesn't include sales to hospitals. However, the drug has just been reclassified by the FDA and put on its list of controlled substances. Beginning in 1981, Darvon prescriptions will be nonrenewable. If negative studies continue to appear, its popularity is likely to plunge.

How to Take Darvon

Take Darvon with water and food. Be sure not to drink any alcoholic beverages when using it, because Darvon in combination with alcohol or tranquilizers can be dangerous. The same is to be said for its interaction with the other mood drugs listed on page 149, as well as with sleeping pills and muscle relaxants. These combinations have been implicated in a number of suicides and accidental deaths.

Codeine

Codeine is a highly regarded painkiller that belongs to the morphine family. Like morphine, it is a natural derivative of opium, the juice of the poppy plant known as *Papaver somniferum* ("the poppy of sleep"). The use of opium as a painkiller was widespread in the Middle Ages and is attested to as far back as 4000 B.C. in the written records of Sumerian physicians.

Far weaker than morphine or Demerol, codeine is not normally considered a dangerous drug. In one study, chronic pain patients given 32 mg. of codeine four times a day (a standard moderate dose) for three months showed no signs of withdrawal when another drug was substituted for the codeine without their knowledge. However, while codeine doesn't usually lead to physical dependence, it can, in people with a tendency to abuse alcohol or other drugs, create a psychological dependence.

Nevertheless, used for pain (and never for depression, which it only compounds), codeine is an excellent analgesic for moderate to severe pain. It can cause tolerance and should be used with care, but if used intermittently it can be taken in quite high doses (to be checked first with your physician, of course). Constipation, nausea, and vomiting are frequently reported side effects. Some people experience euphoria with codeine; others call it "mental clouding" and would rather do without. As with all drugs, *you* are the one to decide if you are benefiting and whether the gains outweigh any negative reactions.

How to Take Codeine

Codeine is prepared in tablets of either 30 or 60 mg. However, it is most frequently prescribed in pre-mixed combinations containing either aspirin or Tylenol. This has both advantages and disadvantages. My own preference is to use codeine alone and, when I need stronger analgesia, to take it with aspirin. Most enlightened doctors will accept that patients should have access to both medications in separate form so that each patient is able to use them according to individual and shifting needs.

The major advantage of a premixed combination is that a simple analgesic (either aspirin or Tylenol) potentiates the effect of codeine. This makes 30 mg. of codeine plus one aspirin tablet more effective for your pain than either 60 mg. of codeine or two aspirin, according to accepted medical practice. Thus, by combining codeine with a simple analgesic, you can slow the rate of tolerance development by using lower doses of codeine.

If you don't need, or can't tolerate, aspirin, you shouldn't be taking a premixed combination that contains it. Take codeine alone, or codeine with acetaminophen (Tylenol). Bear in mind that if you develop tolerance to codeine, you will need to take higher doses of it. In a premixed combination, you will therefore be taking higher doses of aspirin or Tylenol, both of which can have undesirable consequences in the long run.

Codeine should be taken with water or milk and never on an empty stomach. As with the other narcotic analgesics, leave at least an hour on either side free of alcoholic beverages. Codeine can be dangerous in combination with alcohol, tranquilizers, or other mood-altering drugs.

Percodan

The main ingredient in Percodan, which also contains aspirin, phenacetin, and caffeine, is oxycodone, a synthetic drug with a chemical structure similar to morphine. Percodan is a strong painkiller with significant ability to affect perception and mood. As with most other morphine-like agents, reactions to it differ widely. For many people, it is a stimulant, which means that it would not be the drug of choice for nighttime pain. Others are laid so low by its numbing effect that they find it hard to stay awake.

Percodan has a faster onset of action than Darvon or codeine, which may be an advantage if you are in a hurry for relief. On the other hand, if its effect on you is very powerful, you want to be able to stay put once you've taken it. Percodan is not the kind of pill to take as you go out the door or on your way home from work. It can begin to act, subject to individual variation, within fifteen to thirty minutes.

How to Take Percodan

Take Percodan with food in your stomach and an ample swig of milk or water. Alcohol, tranquilizers, and other mood-altering drugs are strictly contraindicated. If gastric irritation is a problem, ask your doctor to switch you to Percocet, which contains Tylenol instead of aspirin.

Talwin

Talwin, like Percodan, is a synthetic agent that was developed for its similarity to morphine in the continuing search for a painkiller with morphine's analgesic strength but without its addictive liability. Since it was first released in 1967, Talwin has taken its place in the standard repertoire of prescription analgesics. Unfortunately, Talwin is neither as effective for severe pain nor as free of side effects as was first believed. A significant number of patients experience frequent nausea and vomiting, as well as hallucinations or an alarming sense of disorientation, which makes this drug less desirable than others for "ambulatory" patients — those who are not confined to bed. On the positive side, Talwin is more powerful than codeine and is slower to build tolerance than Demerol.

How to Take Talwin
Take Talwin with food and water. Alcohol, tranquilizers, and other mood-altering drugs are strictly contraindicated.

Demerol

Demerol is another synthetic narcotic analgesic. Developed in the early 1940s, it is widely, although mistakenly, viewed by both patients and doctors as the "last stop" before morphine. Many doctors shy away from giving Demerol to patients with chronic pain, except in times of acute exacerbation. However, under the proper conditions, people who either cannot tolerate the other narcotic analgesics or get no relief from them may find Demerol a useful drug. As always, the decision rests with you and your physician.

How to Take Demerol

Take Demerol with food and water. Dangerous interactions are the same as for Talwin, *with this important addition:* if you are taking any drug that belongs to the monoamine oxidase (MAO) inhibitor group of antidepressants — including isocarboxazid (Marplan), phenelzine (Nardil), and tranylcypromine (Parnate) — DO NOT TAKE DEMEROL. Severe reactions can occur.

Some Rules of Thumb for Maximizing Drug Effectiveness

- Know the basic facts on any drug you plan to use. Refer to the five-point profile on page 153 if necessary. Remember that your own observations about how a given drug affects you are more important than any standardized description.

- Always choose the smallest effective dose of the weakest drug that works. Don't overshoot the mark. You want to keep tolerance at bay.

- Take painkillers *before* pain becomes excruciating. Holding out until the bitter end makes it harder for a drug to work and can force you to resort to stronger medication when a weaker one might suffice.

- Tolerance to all the narcotic analgesics except Percodan (which already contains aspirin) can be slowed by alternating the drug with either Tylenol or aspirin. For example, instead of taking codeine every four hours, take it every eight hours, with Tylenol or aspirin in between.

- Be sure to take a generous amount of milk or water with all painkillers, both to minimize gastric upset and to speed entry into your digestive tract.

- Save pain medication *for pain only;* if your pain keeps you awake at night, consult your doctor on an appropriate nighttime drug (antihistamines like diphenhydramine [Benadryl] are favored for their low incidence of tolerance buildup and side effects).

- Cigarette smoking may increase the metabolism of most drugs. If you smoke tobacco, you may need to take pain medication more frequently to get the analgesic action you require.

- Be sure you have given a drug a fair trial before switching to another. Sometimes a change in dose (either upward, or downward if you are trying to reduce side effects) can dramatically increase drug effectiveness.

- If you do switch from one pain medication to another, your doctor should prescribe equianalgesic doses. You may be more sensitive to one drug than to another, and you don't want to set yourself up for whopping side effects by taking a larger dose of a drug you've never tried. This means that 2 aspirin tablets provide the same analgesic effect as 30 mg. of codeine or 65 mg. of Darvon or 1 Percodan tablet or 25 mg. of Talwin or 50 mg. of Demerol.

- Remember that painkillers are only part of your repertoire of pain-coping tools. When you can, do without them.

10

Dealing with Doctors

From the doctor's summing up Ivan Ilyich concluded that things were bad, but that for the doctor, and perhaps for everybody else, it was a matter of indifference, though for him it was bad. And this conclusion struck him painfully, arousing in him a great feeling of pity for himself and of bitterness toward the doctor's indifference to a matter of such importance.

He said nothing of this, but rose, placed the doctor's fee on the table, and remarked with a sigh, "We sick people probably often put inappropriate questions. But tell me, in general, is this complaint dangerous, or not?"

The doctor looked at him sternly over his spectacles with one eye, as if to say, "Prisoner, if you will not keep to the questions put to you, I shall be obliged to have you removed from the court."

"I have already told you what I consider necessary and proper. The analysis may show something more." And the doctor bowed.

LEO TOLSTOY,
The Death of Ivan Ilyich

Tolstoy put the final touches on *The Death of Ivan Ilyich* almost a century ago. Medicine has made great strides since then, but the doctor-patient relationship he depicted is as recognizable today as if it had been sketched by a modern novelist. That relationship, already on the skids so many years ago, is now almost universally acknowledged to be in something of a full-fledged crisis. Growing numbers of people are turning away from organized medicine and looking to a broad spectrum of other healers — psychotherapists, acupuncturists, social workers, herbalists, chiropractors, homeopathists — to do what many physicians no longer seem able or willing to do: quite simply, make us feel better.

■ ■ ■

Nowhere, perhaps, has the gap between doctors and patients run so deep — or provoked so much alienation — as between physicians and patients with chronic pain. From opposite sides of a broad, imposing desk we confront each other like two strangers whose words vanish in thin air across a vast abyss. Words are spoken but they aren't heard; a gulf of misunderstanding separates the two opposing sides. Patients with chronic pain strain doctors' scientific knowledge to the breaking point; doctors seem to lack the very quality they find so laudable in us: patience. Our needs are pressing, but long-term; physicians' attention spans are short. Our needs are personal; to many physicians we are just another face, one they sometimes seem to have confused with our disease. And so it goes.

To some degree this split is a case of mutual misunderstanding, a communication problem. It also reflects a growing impatience on the part of many doctors with medical approaches that are neither quick, nor glamorous, nor lucrative.

Since the end of World War II, new technologies, along

with the advent of television, have made heroic medicine a space-age media event. With spectacular acute-care triumphs — cardiac resuscitation, the reattachment of severed limbs, the replacement of organs that were only recently considered irreplaceable — making international reputations and six-figure incomes, there has been a dramatic shift away from lowly general practice, as personified by the stethoscoped family doctor of yesteryear, toward the ready glamour of more rescue-oriented specializations.

To patients with pain, it sometimes seems that fewer and fewer physicians are interested in treating the chronic illnesses that still account for so much human suffering.* You yourself, like one lupus patient I interviewed, may have had the feeling of just not being an interesting enough "case" to command serious medical attention and concern. Of course, many physicians *are* seriously concerned about patients with chronic pain but simply don't know how to help. Doctors whose training increasingly emphasizes total cure may feel unprepared or even inadequate when faced with medical conditions that do not respond to the available techniques. (A number of recent articles in the medical journals indicate that physicians and other health professionals have a poor understanding of basic concepts relating to pain.) Actually, there is a great deal to be said for plain old-fashioned *care*.

Cure vs. Care: Closer Than We Think

Curing any ailment is still the primary goal of medicine, as it should be. But not all the ills that befall us have cures within the grasp of modern medicine, despite its great sophistication. Illnesses such as cancer, arthritis, hypertension,

* Despite the fact that most visits to practicing physicians are not for illnesses that require a specialist, as of 1973 more than 76 percent of American doctors were specialists.

migraine, diabetes, multiple sclerosis, and many other almost certainly involve a whole web of interconnecting causes — including genetic susceptibility, environmental factors, diet, and an individual's general level of resistance to disease. Because of this complexity, what may eventually emerge, rather than a single cure, is the ability to prevent the causing factors from converging in such a way as to produce a particular disease.

Meanwhile, failing a known cure for what we have, optimum care — and optimism — are what we need. Because so little is understood about the dynamics that govern many pain-producing illnesses and about the process of pain itself, the doctor who provides good care — attentive symptomatic treatment along with a shared effort at mobilizing the patient's own healing power — is making a significant contribution toward helping each of us move as close to cure as we can get. The skill involved in awakening "the doctor within each patient," as Dr. Albert Schweitzer called it, is every bit as impressive as that required to revive a heart that has stopped beating. This is particularly important to remember in view of the fact that many serious diseases remit or disappear in ways that surpass present medical understanding. When both physicians and patients realize this, the treatment of chronic illness — and chronic pain — will have made its own spectacular advance.

Bridging the Gap: Why and How

Doctors *can* be more responsive to patient needs and patients *can* have a tremendous impact on defining the kind of relationship they want with doctors. The present gap in communication and understanding is disturbing but not beyond repair. Clearly, medical schools need to redress some of the grievous lacks in their curricula by making such courses as interpersonal dynamics, psychology of illness, and pain management an integral part of every doctor's preparation. But that is *their* problem. *Our* side of the story is figuring out how to deal with doctors more effectively, productively, smoothly, and comfortably. Being a patient doesn't mean being a passive recipient of medical services. On the contrary. The more informed you are, and the more actively you participate in your own care, the more you will be helping your physician help you.

Why Doctors?

Almost everyone requires medical assistance at one time or another, and most people can't afford to bypass the existing health structure. In some cultures the healer may be a shaman or a priest or priestess or a midwife or a sorcerer (all counterparts of Western-defined medical experts), but right now, in our culture, the only officially sanctioned healer is the physician. Since the only services most insurance programs cover are those supplied by physicians or hospital staff, the kinds of treatment you can seek will — unless you have money to spare — be limited to those recognized by the major private carriers or government-run programs (Medicaid, Medicare). This means that you will be dealing with doctors even if only to get beyond them to the many nontraditional treatments — acupuncture, hypnosis, relaxation therapies, biofeedback — that hospitals and clinics around the country are beginning to explore.

■ ■ ■

Whether you are scouting for a new doctor or seeking to improve the relationship you have with your present one, your first priority is to turn your own head around. You need to break the hold of medical intimidation. Almost everyone

I know suffers from what I call medical amnesia. Let's say you enter a doctor's office with five questions. With a little luck you ask three of them, and when you walk out the office door you draw a total blank when you try to remember what was said. This serious problem is a sign of the fear, doubt, and intimidation that grip so many people the minute they step inside a doctor's office.

Down with Intimidation: Why Not Look at It This Way?

When you make an appointment with a new doctor, you're setting up an interview. Who's being interviewed? The doctor. Who's doing the interviewing? You! For what? The job of helping you get better. Of course it's not a one-way proposition. You're offering an interesting position to someone with the imagination and the right scientific background to help *you* do the job. While the suggestions that follow are intended as guidelines for choosing a new physician, they can also help clarify your thoughts regarding the doctor with whom you are already in treatment.

Getting Started

The first step in the right direction is defining:

- what you want in a doctor
- what you can expect from a doctor
- what to look for in a doctor
- when to move on

What You Want in a Doctor

Not everybody is looking for exactly the same kind of doctor-patient relationship. There is no single correct model. Some people want a partnership of equals, others prefer the distance that authority confers. Some patients want to understand the physiology of their illness or condition, while others would rather leave such details to the doctor. But however you define the doctor-patient relationship, you can't choose *not* to participate in it. When you've already got chronic pain, you are already part of it. You can choose to be passive, but there is no question that by becoming an informed, active participant you will receive better-quality care and will probably feel better in the long run. Whether you're looking for a parent figure or a partner or something in between, by extending your sense of *responsibility* to the doctor-patient relationship you are enlisting not only the doctor's energy but your own in improving your health.

What You Can Expect from a Doctor

The most important point to keep in mind is that what doctors need to know about their patients and what patients need to know about themselves involves an *exchange of two related but different bodies of knowledge.* Be prepared for specific, scientific, sometimes personal questions. Remember that the doctor is going to be looking for cause and effect. The doctor's training is *not* in subtleties of dialogue or in the possible emotional reaction you have to your illness and any problems it is causing you. First and foremost in his or her mind is how best to approach your condition with the available treatments. By available treatments, the doctor probably isn't thinking of vitamins, acupuncture, hypnosis, snake venom, or yoga. If these are on *your* mind, you have to speak up and make your interests known.

What to Look For in a Doctor

What can fairly well be said across the board, regardless of your underlying condition, is that you should have a doctor who you feel respects you and is willing to relate to you more or less as you would wish. A sensitive physician knows that people with chronic pain are often anxious regarding their ability to function, maintain their social connections, and survive financially. Such a person should respect your need to ask questions and have those questions answered in terms *you* understand.

The word *doctor* comes from *docere*, the Latin word meaning "to teach." A good doctor should teach you what you need and want to know about the meaning of your condition (how serious it is, whether it is likely to require major changes in your lifestyle, and how long it might persist), as well as explain the available treatments, both nondrug and drug, with information about the possible benefits and disadvantages of each. If a doctor prescribes medication, you should know exactly why a particular drug has been selected, how long you may need to take it, and *how* to take it. Be suspicious of any doctor who suggests the long-term use of tranquilizers or antidepressants for chronic pain. If you have significant anxiety, whether it relates directly to your pain or not, you need to deal with it, not mask it.* You would be wise to get professional counseling and work your problems through instead of covering them up. (See the Coping Resource Guide beginning on page 231.) Finally, your doctor should be someone whose fees you can afford, or one who has a "sliding" fee that will accommodate your budget.

---

* In a report on the effects of such drugs as Valium and Librium on anxiety in a number of different animals — cats, monkeys, dogs, fish, and rats — Dr. Jeffrey A. Gray, of Oxford University, concluded: "Any drug which reduces the experience of anxiety is likely also to reduce one's capacity to develop . . . methods of coping with stress. The brain produces anxiety because anxiety is needed. It cannot be eliminated without paying a price." (*Executive Health*, April 1979.)

When to Move On

If you feel talked down to, slighted, made fun of, humored, overmedicated, or intimidated, you are dealing with the wrong person.* Change doctors and start from scratch.

Preparing for the Appointment

1. **Plan ahead.** Once you've made an appointment, whether with your regular doctor (if you have one) or with somebody new, it is always a good idea to plan ahead. You don't want to go in one more time feeling like a little child and leaving your adult self out in the waiting room. That's the path that leads to medical amnesia.

2. **Make a written record.** I have found it extremely helpful to write out a clear, numbered list of questions on a clean page in my Pain Journal. (This makes sense for phone conversations with doctors, too.) I put the doctor's name and date at the top of the page, and when the visit begins I'm ready to roll.

3. **Get outside support.** If this is a new doctor, or if for any reason the situation feels threatening to you, have a friend or relative go with you for support. If you know someone who has dealt with doctors before, so much the better. A support person not only can make your time in the waiting room more bearable but can usually come with you into the doctor's office at your request. Having someone you trust with you in the inner sanctum can be valuable in three important ways. A support person is reassuring to you; a support person can back you up if you forget an important question or get rattled or upset; and a support person can help you

* Women, see *The Hidden Malpractice* by Gena Corea for a powerful analysis of male doctors' attitudes toward female patients.

evaluate your own impressions once you leave the doctor's office.

4. **Gather histories and documents in advance.** When you make an appointment, ask the doctor or receptionist exactly what you should bring along. Most doctors seeing you for the first time will want a complete copy of your medical record so they can see exactly what tests you've had, and where, as well as what diagnosis has been made and what treatment you've received to date. Your Medical History on pages 58–59 and your Pain Inventory, page 61, will be useful here.

5. **Clarify your thoughts.** If you aren't clear about what you want to say, use your Pain Journal to write an imaginary letter to the doctor. Get out your feelings and your fears; clear questions will emerge from those.

> "Dear Doctor, I suffer from hope, and from modesty, and I ask you as few questions as I can."
>
> Colette

In the Waiting Room

If possible, bring something to do — a book or magazine to read, a crossword puzzle, a piece of clay to model, or a pad to doodle on. You've probably been to enough doctors by now to know that you are going to have to *wait*. That's what waiting rooms are for, isn't it? There's no point in chewing your nails because you're not enticed by last year's *Lettuce Growers' Magazine* or *Tropical Fish Quarterly*.

This is a good time to write in your Pain Journal. You can go over your questions, clear your head, and express any lingering anxieties. *Aikido* can be a handy concept here too. Let yourself feel the centered strength of your *ki* as you take a few deep breaths and imagine yourself stepping into the doctor's office with all your wits about you. What you want is to stay in touch with the calm at the center of the storm, so that you aren't thrown by any intimidating energy that comes your way. If you give yourself a chance to get centered before your name is called, you'll be clear-minded and clear-spoken when you get inside.

In the Doctor's Office

In my own experience, I've found it very helpful to begin an initial meeting by acknowledging what one woman I interviewed called "the ego wound of the doctor": the sense of failure that so often afflicts doctors and other health practitioners who treat chronic problems, particularly pain.

"I know it's not easy to deal with this sort of thing," you might say. "In fact, it might be almost as hard for you as the doctor as it is for me as the patient." A little compassion goes a long way toward opening the channels of communication. "Naturally I don't expect miracles. But I'd like to know how you would approach my case and whether you think we could work together." A similar tack can be used with a doctor you already know: "I'd like to know whether it might be a good idea to try X or Y. I'm very interested in seeing how it would affect me, and I wonder what your thinking is."

As soon as you've put out a simple opening statement, be sure to give the doctor a chance to respond. Listen well, and jot down any impressions you don't want to forget. The doctor may ask you to tell "how it all began," or to describe your pain in very precise, anatomical terms. This information is essential in order for him or her to get a sense of how to proceed. If you're nervous or anxious or close to tears, say so. Don't wait for the emotions to pile up. Pain compounders are pain compounders, even in a doctor's office. Keep your message clear. The more straightforward you can be about what you're looking for and how you feel, both physically and emotionally, the more you give the doctor to respond to and the faster you will get a sense of him or her. When you lay your cards on the table, the doctor has to do the same.

Some doctors will be put off by this approach and will dismiss you as one more "doctor-shopper." What you have to do is remember what you're doing: interviewing. This isn't a one-time visit we're talking about now. This is the person you want to be able to call on through thick and thin — infrequently, you hope, but for however long your pain presents a problem. If you notice signs of impatience, boredom, or exasperation, don't ignore them. You might try an approach along the lines of "I get the feeling you're not really interested in working with me, doctor. Am I right?" Not many doctors are used to being leveled with. What you want is not so much to walk out of there with a prescription in your fist as to ask good questions, listen well, and get a sense of your prospective physician. Be sure that you ask all the questions on your list and that you understand all the answers. Write them down. Take your time.

After you've asked all your questions, if a friend or relative has come into the office with you, you might want to turn to him or her and say, "Well, I think that just about covers everything we had in mind, doesn't it?" That way your backup person can ask any questions you may have overlooked or ask for clarification of a point you may have missed. Any doctor who objects to this dynamic is not the right man or woman for the job.

Like any other skill, learning to deal with doctors takes practice and perseverance. It's not easy to reverse the pervasive conditioning that tells you you're a victim if you're sick. You may not succeed on the first try. Stay with your quest. Don't settle for someone who doesn't feel right to you. Be tough, keep trying, and you *will* find a doctor you can trust. You'll know it was worth it when you're able to say, like one man I interviewed, "I'm no longer a spectator of my own life; I'm a participant." You'll also have the satisfaction of being a participant in something larger than your own life: the transformation of the way medicine is being practiced today.

■ 11

Pain-Free Relating: Spouses, Lovers, Friends, and Others

Those who do not feel pain seldom think that it is felt.
SAMUEL JOHNSON

"Pain is something you can't share. No matter how graphically you attempt to describe it, it's a personal experience." — Person with chronic pain

"It gets very confusing relating to the person you thought you were relating to. Whatever you're giving isn't being received." — Lover of person with chronic pain

Living with chronic pain is a subtle, ever-changing, continuously challenging process. It demands the most of our capacity to know ourselves, to be honest with ourselves, and, most important of all, to limit ourselves while living with the fullest sense of possibility. This complicated tension between limit and possibility is with us day in and day out. It is what can make chronic pain so frustrating for some and so ultimately life-enhancing for others. If it is hard for us — who, after all, inhabit our own bodies — think how complicated it becomes when someone else enters the picture. To someone on the "outside," our omnipresent inner guest — throbbing, burning, pounding, knifing — is usually invisible.

Other people just don't seem to understand what chronic pain is all about. As one man put it, "They see me up and around and they think it's over and done, which isn't the case at all." A woman with sciatic pain from a botched injection described the well-meaning neighbors who, knowing her love of music, repeatedly called her on an hour's notice with an offer of tickets to the opera. "They know I can't sit through even a short concert because of my back," Sonia said, "but they just can't accept it. So they keep offering me tickets. I resent like crazy having to remind them time after time that there are certain things I just can't do."

Chronic pain makes "outsiders" extremely uncomfortable. They don't want to acknowledge the existence of something they feel they can't do anything about. A good friend of mine calls me up and says, "Hi, how are you — fine?" His greeting tells me that he doesn't want to know. The other side of this particular coin is what happens when friends or kin focus on your health to the exclusion of all else. Colette described this situation:

> Our closest friends . . . write us letters with a maximum of reserve and a minimum of news about themselves, remaining silent about their own troubles and concerned entirely with ours — let me particularize and say "with me" and my arthritis: they have discovered an osteopath who . . . a radiologist whom they . . . They quote the case of a miraculous cure, a thermal spring where . . .
>
> This has the immediate effect of bringing out the worst in my character, since I had anticipated reading

an account of their journey, the events of their stay, the exact number of teeth cut by their small daughter, the exact height of the floods in their district — in short, their news. Have none of my friends, my dearest friend included, the least idea of what interests me?

Still another situation is the "credibility gap" that can arise when friends assume that because they can't *see* your pain it isn't there. Unless your face turns ashen or you roll your eyes, they don't believe you really hurt. This may be the most maddening attitude of all for those of us who try not to show our suffering. One man I interviewed felt betrayed by friends who completely misinterpreted his need to "lie around":

> "Visually, nothing looked like I was hurting. No blood, no guts . . . I spent the whole summer on my back and everybody thought I was being lazy. No one really believed that I had physical pain."

Situations like these reinforce the "damned if you do, damned if you don't" feeling that makes it so difficult to deal with others when you have chronic pain. If you *do* let people know when you're feeling bad and what your limitations are, they have a hard time hearing it and often don't believe you. Telling them once doesn't seem to be enough, which means you're constantly being forced to remind everyone — and be reminded yourself — of how sick you are and what your limitations are. On the other hand, if you *don't* let people know what's going on, they assume you're fine, which can lead to all sorts of misunderstandings:

> "I wouldn't have asked you to carry the groceries if I had realized you were feeling that bad."
> "I figured you would know I was in lousy shape since I was up all night."
> "I didn't know you were up all night."
> "Didn't you hear me moving around?"

Either way, you feel cornered by your pain, which gives you no respite from the subtleties of relating to friends and loved ones. If only people would understand that it's not just the pain that's so hard to take but the fact of having to confront all these ongoing uncertainties about how to cope! Their inability to understand this — the complexity of the chronic pain experience — makes us feel as if a wall of incomprehension had been thrown up between us and the very people we most need to have understand us.

The whole situation is compounded by the fact that we are all under the sway of two solidly entrenched beliefs: (1) that people in pain shouldn't talk about their suffering and other people shouldn't ask, and (2) that other people should be sensitive enough to know when we're in pain, even when we're doing our best to cover it up, and should intuitively understand what we can and cannot do; we shouldn't have to tell them.

Try to imagine being strapped into a straightjacket and having a gag stuffed into your mouth at a time when you're already under stress and in need of close connections with friends and family. This is precisely the effect of the laws of silence we allow to rule our lives. Thanks to them, people in pain are enveloped in a sort of pain mystique.

The Pain Mystique

You don't have to go to law school to learn the rules. In *Medical Nemesis* the presumably enlightened Ivan Illich states with no hesitation: "My compassion is not the same for someone who himself says that he suffers as it is for someone who is said to suffer." Basically, this attitude toward pain in relation to others is an extension of the prevailing cultural-religious view that governs our own responses to pain. If for sufferers the greatest virtue lies in bearing pain with dignity and strength, then for others it lies in treating us with awed compassion when we are most successful in our role.

This attitude hurts everyone, not just those of us in pain but everyone around us. First of all, it makes us feel inadequate, lonely, and unique when in reality we are none of these — not when there are 40 million of us in the United States. Secondly, it gives other people, especially those we are closest to and who care about us most, no way of knowing how we are really feeling and no hint of how to relate to us when we are in pain. We disappear behind the pain mystique as if we had suddenly been swallowed up by an impenetrable mist.

"Outsiders" may occasionally wonder what it's like to live with so much pain, but they aren't supposed to ask and we aren't supposed to tell. The mystique begins when they start imagining how "brave" we are, and how "magnificently" we're handling everything. If they knew what was really going on inside us, they'd have fewer illusions.

When you're living through one of life's most challenging experiences you can't afford the guessing games, charades, and piled-up tensions that inevitably accompany the pain mystique. You can't afford them because you pay with pain, mental anguish, and, if matters get out of hand, sometimes even the desertion of friends and loved ones who can't cope with the strain.

See What I Mean?
I call the press agent of a famous movie star who is known to suffer from severe arthritis. I explain that I am writing a self-help book on pain and ask whether she thinks he might be willing to be interviewed.

"Well," she begins, "he doesn't like to talk about his own anguish. He's a very brave man."

"Still," I persist, "I'd be fascinated to know what he thinks about pain and how he deals with it."

"I'll speak to him," she assures me. "I doubt he'll agree to do it. But if you could get him to open up, I'm sure he could be very inspirational."

Only after I had hung up the phone did I realize that this was a classic conversation about pain — from the outside looking in. The actor in pain was an object of awe, a *brave* sufferer who kept his *anguish* admirably quiet. If I could lure him out from behind his protective screen (the pain mystique), he would no doubt be *inspirational*. Poor man, I thought. That's a hard role to play, even for an actor!

Off With the Veil

By learning to express your feelings in a clear, simple, undemanding way, you can begin to emerge from under wraps. This entails three important realizations:

- You can't expect other people to read your mind.
- By letting other people know what pain means and has meant to you, you will immediately reduce tensions a thousandfold.
- There is an enormous difference between talking and complaining.

Talking vs. Complaining

For many people the idea of talking about their pain seems disgraceful as well as risky. "I don't want to burden them with my troubles" and "People get tired of hearing about it" were typical responses among the men and women I interviewed. Complaining does get to be a burden. Because it alienates people, you also run the risk of losing their friendship or even their love. But talking and complaining are not the same. If more people realized this, they wouldn't censor their need to talk.

Talking is a form of communication. Complaining isn't. Complaining is a poor substitute for throwing a tantrum or blowing your stack. It is usually the result of too much silence and too little talking. There's nothing wrong with complaining once in a while, just so long as you realize what you're doing. Complaining doesn't go anywhere; it uses words to go around and around — like a smoke ring. You may derive a certain satisfaction from complaining if your words bring you a sympathetic nod or a pat on the back, but you won't learn anything. All you hear when you complain is the sound of your own voice.

Talking is another story. Talking is open-ended; it moves toward someone else, creating the possibility of dialogue. You never know where it will lead, because when you ask questions, you can't predict how another person will respond. Imagine asking a good friend or someone you love how *they* feel when you're in pain. You're acknowledging *their* pain — the pain of onlookers — and opening up a whole process of communication that can take you and your companion to a level of understanding complaining never dreamt of.

The Return of the Three R's

If open-ended talking becomes a regular part of your coping repertoire, you won't be peering at your friends and family through the veil of the pain mystique. I know of no better tool for navigating a safe passage out of the mists than the three-point compass you already have at hand: *recognition, responsibility,* and *receptivity.*

Recognition

You almost always have a choice as to whether or not to express your suffering to others. For your own sake it's important to be aware of when you are feeling pain and why, so that you can respond with the full array of coping skills you've already learned. When other people are involved, recognition can help you see the kinds of choices you are making in the way you relate to them. Recognition always gives you more choices than you thought you had.

One man with frequent cluster headaches told me:

> "When I get a bad headache at work I never say anything. I get very tense but I feel that I have to keep on working because everyone else is working so hard. I feel embarrassed to say I need a break. When I get home I take it all out on my wife. I feel really bad about this, because if I could be more honest and let off some of the pressure at work, I probably wouldn't be in so much pain by the end of the day."

As soon as he said this, Jay realized that the answer to his problem lay in his own words. The potential embarrassment of mentioning his pain at work was really minor compared with the effect his held-in tension was having on his wife. He realized he would be much happier at home by saying a few simple words at work: "I need five minutes to cool out. My head is splitting." Not everyone can take a break easily, but five minutes is usually within reach on almost any job.

Another man used recognition to define needs he hadn't been aware of. After two lonely hospitalizations for operations on his ulcerated leg, he realized that his superman image had kept his friends away. "I finally learned," he said, "that it was important that I have visitors, it was important that I have phone calls, and it was important that I get cards — it really gives you the feeling that you're not alone. I also learned to put out my need and not expect them to know it without my saying it."

Recognition can also help you figure out where certain problems are coming from. Not all the tensions in your dealings with other people have to do with pain. In fact, most don't. A brusque bank teller will be just as brusque whether you're in pain or not. All kinds of situations take their toll on us now just as they did before. You may have had problems with your boss long before your back went haywire. Or your teenage kids may have been a handful even then. If you think about it, before you were even in the hospital, inflation was beginning to eat into your choice of menus and strain the atmosphere at meals.

In all these situations, recognition can help you locate the source of your reactions and feelings. The more you can separate your pain from those aspects of your life it has nothing to do with, the freer you will be to deal with pain as befits pain and the other issues in the ways that are appropriate to them.

Responsibility

Even when you're alone it's hard to find the right balance between doing as much as you can and not doing too much. The same holds true when you're in company. People tend to form a single conception of what you can or cannot do and then stick with it forever after. They may overestimate or underestimate your ability to do certain things at certain times.

Most people aren't stupid or insensitive. But given the fluctuations characteristic of most chronic pain, you have to tell them how you're feeling at the moment or take the consequences. They can't possibly know that the three blocks you walked yesterday seem like an impossible mile today. Or that standing at the bus stop would be worse than walking two blocks to the subway. Or that just this once you'd be glad to walk instead of taking the bus because you want the air or the company. No one should be expected to puzzle out all the tiny chips of information you're juggling in your mind. I've had the experience myself of being with a group of people and managing to hold my own despite intense pain and then, when some distant destination was proposed, having to say, "I don't think I can make it that far." "Why — are you in pain?" my friends ask in surprise. To someone who hasn't lived with pain for a long time, it is inconceivable that a person could appear quite calm — even carry on an animated conversation — and still be in a lot of pain. *You* have to give the cues.

Covering Up: How Much Is OK?

There are certain situations where you will be in pain and for any number of reasons not want to have it show or be a topic of conversation. I remember the first time I consciously covered up my pain. I was meeting friends from out of town who knew about my illness. The arrangement, made several weeks ahead, was to meet them at a restaurant along with several other people I didn't know. When the day of our dinner came along, I was feeling terrible, but this was my only chance to see my friends for a whole year. I decided to go anyway and not mention anything about my health. Before leaving the house I wrote in my Pain Journal, "This is the first time I've gone ahead with plans to see friends when I was feeling awful. It's my choice: these are friends I want to see, not people I want to share my pain with!"

I evaluated the evening on my way home: "In terms of what I set out to do, success. I'm glad I went. I was in pain a lot of the time, but it wasn't an 'issue' because I had defined the evening in other terms."

My own rule of thumb about covering up is that it's all right to pull a fast one on others but it's not all right to pull one on yourself. You need to be in touch with what your body is telling you if your coverup is going to be healthy.

Recognition is the word to keep in mind.

This passage from *The Blue Lantern* gives us a glimpse of the majesty and sense of humor that Colette maintained while *knowingly* covering up her pain: "As for the stairs, their descent is not a matter of humiliation and guile: for when a stranger passes, do I not stop and, standing still, pretend to be putting on a glove or fumbling in my bag! Once the stranger is safely out of the way, I laugh at myself and my old woman's wiles."

Another part of taking responsibility for how you deal with pain in social situations involves doing what you need to do for your pain before it gets to the point where you are indirectly (and perhaps unconsciously) manipulating other people into telling you to sit down, lie down, or take your medicine. When you put others in the position of policing you, you're setting up a situation where people begin to equate you with your pain.

Separating Yourself from Your Pain

"You are *not* your pain. Overwhelming as your pain may be, it is only one part of your whole life." Remember? If you don't take responsibility for listening to what your pain is asking for, the effects spill over onto everyone around you. When the only self you're putting on view is your self-in-pain, people *do* tend to move on. You want to make it clear that you know the difference between having pain become your whole identity and having it be a part of you that has to be accepted.

Receptivity

The art of listening is as important in relation to others as it is in relation to yourself. The idea is to keep your ear tuned to the limits of possibility. If you can't go to the beach or climb the bleachers with family and friends, you can all sit down together and figure out a new way to enjoy your leisure time together. There is always a new way of approaching even a severely disabling situation. If *you* don't think of it, maybe someone else will. On this score, people with chronic pain may have to do a little educating of those "outsiders" whose advice becomes a burden instead of being helpful. Anyone can be told (gently and with tact) that there's a tremendous difference between advice and interest. By making that distinction, you will find it easier to be receptive to what others have to offer.

Interest vs. Advice

Chronic pain makes many people so uneasy that they either block it out completely (like Sonia's well-meaning neighbors with their offers of last-minute tickets to the opera) or flood you with advice about fantastic doctors, treatments, ointments, articles, clinics, and appointments. Most advice is certainly well meant. But that doesn't mean it's well received by us, or that it should be. One woman with chronic pain from a broken hip told me, "Advice really wears you down. It just reinforces that people see you only in terms of your pain."

People don't like to see someone who isn't getting better. Advice fills the space between them and you and makes them feel they're doing something. Its main function is to relieve *their* sense of impotence. What it does to you is not so nice. When people give advice there is almost always an underlying message that says, "If you don't try this, then you haven't done everything you could to get better." Advice judges you and puts you on the spot while it lets the other person off the hook. (Maybe once you try X or Y you'll be better, and then they won't have to face the reality of chronic pain.) Advice from others, like complaining from us, is not a very useful form of communication. It is actually a poor substitute for interest.

Interest is a question: "How are you?" Not mechanically, but "I really want to know how you're doing." Interest asks instead of judging. "What else is happening in your life? Does it bother you if I ask about your health? If I hear of a good doctor, should I let you know? What can I do to help?" Interest makes a genuine bridge between the person who cares and the person with chronic pain. Most importantly, interest gives *you* the chance to help friends and family overcome feelings of impotence in the face of chronic pain. There are many ways they can help you besides giving you advice. One of the most important is to relate to you as a person — not see just your pain. Other assistance will depend on the extent to which you choose to involve friends, family, and neighbors with any day-to-day requirements of your pain.

Many of the people I interviewed for this book didn't want to make their pain the subject of frequent discussion with family and friends. The wish most often expressed was for others to "understand what this has meant in my life without my having to remind them again and again." If this is how you feel, sometimes one good straight talk with those you are closest to is all you need; you can explain that from then on, you'll give the cues if there are any changes that require further conversation. It's also important to remember that the people who are closest to you experience their own kind of pain. It is both hard and disturbing to see a loved one suffer. They may need recognition from *you*, acknowledgment of the problems that invariably affect any relationship where pain is a hidden partner. If you can let them know that you are aware of this dimension, too, you will have gone a long way toward clearing the air.*

* Not everyone finds this sort of discussion easy; by showing this chapter to those who matter in your life, you may find it easier to broach the subject and begin to open the channels of communication.

Asking for Help

It's wonderful to be independent, but if your pain or ill health seriously interferes with your ability to shop, cook, get to a health care facility, or keep up your contacts with the outside world, it's important to be able to ask for help. From my own experience I know that this is not an easy lesson to learn, particularly since chronic pain disrupts one of the most important rhythms of our lives, the natural give-and-take of reciprocal arrangements. It's hard to ask for help when you feel you have no way of returning the favor. Being unable to give is a great deprivation. It is also an unnecessary one. No matter what your condition is, there are always ways in which you can give to those around you.

Give-and-Take

Our usual expectation is to repay most favors in kind: "If you take the kids to the swimming meet, I'll pick them up." If your kids always need a ride and you can never do the picking up, you're left with the feeling that you owe more than you can pay. If someone gives you a ride to the doctor once, it's fine, but if you need a lift every week, the sense of dependency begins to get uncomfortable. Naturally, you don't have to return every favor with an immediate response. But in the context of an ongoing arrangement (the friend who shops for you, the in-laws who take your child somewhere special every Sunday afternoon), it's important to make room for your own giving.

You know yourself. You know what you can do. On your better days you may be able to reciprocate, if not in kind, at least in character. If you have crafts skills, you may be able to repair a broken chair for the next-door neighbors who bring in your mail, or hem a skirt, or make a leather wallet or a weaving. You can coach the nephew who's behind in math or teach a friend to type or use a camera. Sharing your creativity and know-how is a wonderful way to show appreciation to the people who help you out. If you're home a lot, even if you have difficulty getting around, you can provide important reassurance to a working mother who needs someone she can count on in a pinch — if, say, her child is sent home sick from school or in an emergency. You may not be able to get down on the floor and play jacks or hide-and-seek, but you can read the child a story or tell jokes until your friend arrives. All these ways of helping help you too. They keep you connected to your giving self, which is a vital part of your own health.

Spouses and Lovers

There is no doubt about it; chronic pain puts a tremendous strain on any intimate relationship. Everyone I interviewed was well aware of this and deeply troubled by it.

Chronic pain almost always brings with it worry, financial strain, and uncertainty about every kind of plan, from day-to-day social arrangements to such long-term issues as vacation dates, your or your mate's ability to take a better job in another neighborhood or town, and so on. Any relationship is bound to suffer when that triple bundle suddenly arrives on the doorstep. In the months following the onset of chronic pain a great adjustment must be made by both members of a couple. In a sense the path is clearer for the one with pain: this is, after all, your own life you are straightening out. The other person's role is not so easily defined. If matters were already rocky between you, there may well be two sets of questions in his or her mind: how can I help? and do I want to help or do I want to get out while the getting is good?

Any preexisting problems are sure to become exacerbated. Household chores take on a new significance. When one person is either no longer able, or temporarily unable, to perform certain tasks (anything from dumping the garbage to stoking the stove to cooking, shopping, or making the bed), the equilibrium of the relationship is thrown off. Normally, no single one of these daily activities makes or breaks a relationship, but in the context of chronic pain a minor change can affect both partners' sense of identity. When Paul spoke of not being able to carry his own groceries, his feelings actually went much deeper:

> "I'm very self-conscious and apprehensive about my capabilities. Before I had this problem I knew that my ace in the hole was that I could always work harder. Now, if things don't work I'm not going to jump in and save the day. I'm limited. Physically limited to what I can do."

Feelings like these can lead to an overall sense of neediness that humiliates the person with chronic pain and may antagonize his or her partner:

> "I need assurance that it's all going to work out, and that I'm not alone in this. People need to be more understanding of what the condition really involves (debt, reduced earning power, depression)."

> "I just wish my wife would realize that I don't want sympathy. I need her to be patient and to accept my moodiness. I guess I need to feel that she still believes in me."

Our needs for understanding and encouragement are real. But not all couples are equally able to absorb the shock waves that result from an experience so consistently demanding as chronic pain. "What you have to realize," one man told me, "is that pain is like a magnifying glass. It doesn't change the original dynamic, it just blows it up. You get an eight-by-ten-inch enlargement instead of a tiny negative, but the picture is the same." Realizing this may be the key to saving a relationship that seems threatened by chronic pain. Most couples tend to focus only on the pain as the root of all their troubles. By getting to work on the problems that were there before the pain, you may find that if those can be worked out, both you and your spouse or lover are more able to confront the issues that result directly from your pain. Couple counseling or short-term psychotherapy is probably a good idea in such a situation.

It's also important not to put all your eggs in one basket. If your needs are focused exclusively on the person with whom you share your life, you may truly be asking for more than anyone can give. If the person you love knows that you are able to discuss some of your problems with close friends, other family members, a trusted member of the clergy, or a counselor, it may ease some of the sense of having to be your only support in times of trouble. As the lover of a woman with chronic pain observed, "The person in pain has to be willing to share the ownership of the illness or condition." The more you reach out, the richer your relationship will be. After all, you don't want pain to be the center of attraction between you and your love.

Lovemaking
Sexual problems as the result of pain are extremely common. They most often occur for one of the following reasons:

- Loss of sexual desire or function due to medication
- Increase in pain during lovemaking, attributable to certain movements or positions
- Diminished sense of personal attractiveness due to disability or pain

If you are experiencing a loss of sexual desire or have become impotent or nonorgasmic, you should, according to Dr. James F. Fries, director of the Stanford Arthritis Clinic, "suspect any drug and talk with your doctor about it." If a drug is causing sexual problems, your doctor should be able to find you a better substitute.

If lovemaking itself brings on or increases pain, you may want to try different positions that put less strain on the affected parts of your body. Sometimes cushions can improve the situation, but it is probably a good idea to get specific suggestions from your doctor or a trained physical therapist or person knowledgeable about body movement, such as a dancer.

If you are experiencing feelings of "unsexiness" because of your pain and any related disability, you may find that even when you're not at your most radiant or vibrant, lovemaking can be a very satisfying turnaround of pain energy. One woman told me that although she feels less like initiating sex when she's in pain, "once it's underway, it's enormously healing. I always felt I had to have all that energy before making love," she continued, "or else I didn't want to. Now I've learned that I can draw on sex *for* energy, which is a wonderful discovery."

12

Coping with Setbacks

> You cannot step twice into the same river, for other
> waters and yet others go ever flowing on.
> ### HERACLITUS

> Reverse cannot befall
> That fine Prosperity
> Whose Sources are interior —
> ### EMILY DICKINSON

One of the built-in frustrations with chronic pain is that
your progress on the "path" doesn't always follow a straight
line. Setbacks can and do occur. Chronic pain, after all, is
chronic — it exists over time. Most chronic illnesses and
many injuries (not all) affect your body differently at different times. The pain of some conditions can all but disappear
for weeks, months, or even years at a time, only to resurface
with a violence you thought you'd finally left behind.

There's also another kind of setback: a setback in your
ability to cope. You may be going strong for a couple of
weeks or months and then suddenly feel overwhelmed by
pain you thought you had under control. All kinds of things

can throw you off, from a bad cold to the threat of layoffs where you work.

How you react to a setback of either type can make all the difference between whether you continue on the path to pain control or stay stranded in the middle of the road.

Naturally, you can't spend your time worrying about what you're going to do when a setback hits. If you're doing better and feeling better, enjoy it to the hilt. It does make sense, though, to be aware from the beginning that *setbacks in no way change the basic direction of your path*. The path to pain control is a path you are on through thick and thin, good times and bad. It is your path to make and your path to follow. If it takes you through a patch of brambles, it will also lead you to a clearing. If you panic you can lose your way. But if you listen to the voice within you — your coping self — the skills you have learned in the course of this book will see you through.

A Setback in Your Pain

It is particularly frustrating to be faced with a setback in your pain just when you begin to gain a modicum of control and feel a whole new sense of possibility enter your life. When a setback follows on the heels of satisfying progress, it's very easy to slip back into old ways of thinking and reacting. This is the time to remember that chronic pain is a formidable, complicated process and that you are most in control when you fight it least. The first lesson in lifesaving is to tell the victim to stop thrashing and let the water carry the body's weight. When you learn to drive, you learn to turn the wheels in the direction of a skid. The same wisdom holds with pain. If you stay calm and don't slam on the brakes, you'll find, in the words of poet Anita Barrow, "that what you have come to is only a halt."

Getting Back on Track

You may be at a halt, but you don't want to stay there. Mentally, *aikido* can help you swoop right in and meet this new wave of pain halfway. "Oh no you don't," you're thinking to yourself, as you immediately begin to chart your course for coping.

The first item on your list is how you immediately respond to the physical pain. Is this a turn of events that warrants medical attention? Is it a sign that you've been overdoing things? What can you do to ease up right away? These are questions only you can answer, depending on the precise nature of your pain or condition. Whatever you have to do to stop this pain from settling in for a long winter, do. Do it immediately, not tomorrow.

The next step is to deal with your emotional response. Pain compounders will be serious contenders for the job of accompanying your setback all along the way. Anger, self-pity, and depression are practically inevitable reactions to a major setback in your health. Acknowledge them, greet them, let them be. Recognition is your ally. Before you can take responsibility for coping with a setback, you have to pass through recognition. It's like going through neutral when you shift gears in a car. You may find it helpful to express your first reactions in your Pain Journal. The more you deal with them early on, the less they will undermine you as you continue on the path.

The third part of your course is to plan a full-scale *aikido* response to turn the setback's energy around:

What you want to do is gather the intensity of your response and with a flick of your wrist redirect it — toward the good friends whose company you value and toward the activities that hold your greatest interest. *Outreach* is the key word to keep you moving in the right direction.

Your Pain Is Not the Same This Time Around

Each time your pain returns, it is different. Why? Because you yourself are different. That's what Heraclitus meant about not stepping twice into the same river. No matter how familiar your pain feels, it is not the same as last time. A different you is feeling it. Since the last time around, you've learned a whole new repertoire of skills for coping. And each time you're faced with a setback, you will have changed since the last one. It's important to be aware of how far you've traveled, because a setback can make you lose sight of all the gains you've made. By recording your reactions in your trusty Pain Journal, you'll be able to watch the way you're responding and catch yourself if you begin to stray off the path. The following extracts from my own journal were written about a year apart when severe pain returned after a long remission. As you can see, I learned a lot in the twelve months between them.

> I feel the chains holding me down, the heavy door swing shut. Back in the pit — pain. I suppose I should be grateful for three months so relatively free of pain. I *am* grateful. But I don't want this! Look how I'm talking — as if I expect to be in pain for the next six months!

> The pain is back. First reactions — disbelief, anger, disappointment. Why does this have to happen to me? Right away I felt that sinking feeling in my stomach, like it's all over. It will be if I think of it that way. But this is a new time around, and I can choose to do it

differently. I know exactly what I have to do. Put my whole pain "apparatus" into gear. My body is making it very easy for me by spelling out its message loud and clear. I don't have someone else's body; I have this one, so this is the one I have to pay attention to. Just because I'm in pain again doesn't mean I have to lose either my new higher spirits or my momentum. My identity is absolutely free to float right over the pain and go its sane, merry way. I don't have to feel compromised, defeated, humiliated, etc. I just have to listen and do the things I know perfectly well now how to do.

A Setback in Your Ability to Cope

When pain goes on day after day, the going can get rough. It's easy to get stuck in patterns of reacting that work for a while and suddenly go bust. It's not your fault. Sometimes the path seems laid out before you and all you have to do is walk. But the day can come when it takes a turn uphill. The going gets slower and you feel yourself running out of steam. Your old tricks aren't working and defeat creeps in. At such a moment you may even slip, just as you might climbing a mountain. This is the time to remember, as you would with a setback in your pain, that coping with chronic pain is a difficult, demanding process and that you are most in control when you fight it least. If you slip, sit down. Dust yourself off and look around. Give yourself a chance to get your bearings before you resume your journey. If you do, you may find that the path isn't half as steep when you get back on your feet.

Getting Your Bearings

You're sitting down, not lying down. There's a tremendous difference. You're not defeated, you're just momentarily winded. To get your bearings at a time like this, you need to catch your breath and draw deeply on what you already know. When Emily Dickinson wrote of "that fine Prosperity whose Sources are interior," she was referring to the inner strengths and rich reserves of creativity we all can learn to mine in our own depths.

Slow motion is the best speed for your initial response. By now you have a whole repertoire of pain coping skills. Are you somewhere where you can relax and take half an hour for yourself? Wherever you are, get into a comfortable position and let your mind skim over all the techniques you have learned. There is probably one approach that you've found useful over and over again. It may be an image you've been relying on for years, or a specific technique you learned from this book. It may be a deep breathing exercise or meditation or just closing your eyes and letting your thoughts wander to memories — or fantasies — of some beautiful place.* By relaxing instead of snapping back to action, you give yourself a chance to get centered again and find the flow of energy you need for coping in the "storm" of chronic pain. You want to begin to unwind the coil of defeatism and turn it around.

Seeing from the Eye of the Storm

When you're relaxed, you're in a good position to look back on the days and weeks leading up to your setback. Let

* If nothing comes to mind, turn to the Pain Emergency Kit on pages 209–26.

recognition be your guide. Without judging, you want to look from the eye of the storm, noticing the tensions that have been building up. Coping with chronic pain is not an isolated process; if you've been having setbacks in other areas of your life, they are bound to affect your ability to handle pain. What emotions surface as you think back on your recent past? Notice them, and take note of the specific pain compounders that are pulling you down. By dealing with them now, you'll find your feet much lighter on the ground when you resume your journey.

Replenishing Your Inner Prosperity

Pain seems new every day. There's that sense of alarm that's so hard to shake even when you know you're not in danger. Even so, it's very easy to be lulled into coping with your pain the same way day after day. Sometimes familiar approaches keep working. But because *you* are always changing, it's more often true that your techniques for coping have to change too. Pain keeps you on your toes.

How have you been dealing with your pain? What are your inner riches? When the path to pain control takes a sharp turn uphill, you're getting a very clear message. Listen. Look back at the lists you made on page 108 and the short-term goals you set out on page 146. When your response to pain becomes habitual, you're no longer listening for the possible. This is the time to fine-tune your awareness of the many avenues toward painlessness you have yet to explore. Perhaps one phone call can link you up to an activity or friendship you've had in mind for months. You might want to reread Chapters 6 and 7 to restore your sense of how to energize the turnaround. The key, as you'll remember, is transformation: turning pain energy into life energy. You can do it now; you've done it before.

It's important to remember to keep your expectations optimistic *and* realistic. Sometimes people run into a setback simply because they lose sight of the nature of chronic pain. A few triumphs can seduce you back into expecting total control. Part of learning to live with chronic pain is knowing — not necessarily liking, but knowing — that there may be times when despite your best efforts, your pain is strong. A certain amount of pain may have to be part of a part of your life. By reviewing and renewing your response to that fact, you will return to the process of coping revitalized and ready for the road.

Beginner's Mind

A new start gives you the chance to strip down to essentials and refocus your vision of the path to pain control. But beginning again doesn't mean beginning with nothing. In the words of Shunryu Suzuki, "In the beginner's mind there are many possibilities; in the expert's mind there are few."

PART IV

Pain Emergency Kit

Pain Emergency Kit

The relaxation and visualization techniques in this section are for those times when nothing else seems to work — late at night when pain is keeping you from sleeping, at work when pain is interfering with your ability to concentrate, or in any number of situations where your usual approach to pain hasn't done the trick. All of them are simple and require only a few minutes of your time. They can be slipped into your life at almost any point throughout the day, whether you're alone or in a room full of people. These techniques can be used in conjunction with pain medication. They are also extremely useful for getting through short-term acute pain situations such as dental work or hospital procedures in which there is a degree of discomfort and anxiety.

Relaxation and visualization techniques aren't lifesavers you can just grab on to whenever the going gets rough. It's important to practice them. One good way of doing this is to incorporate them into a morning ritual that will help you start each day with a relaxed, recentered commitment to staying on the path to pain control. That way the special skills and tricks of this Pain Emergency Kit will be there for you when you really need them for pain.

This section is intended for Browsing. Read through once just to get a sense of the full spectrum of suggestions, letting your eye take in those techniques that particularly appeal to you at first glance. At some point in the next few days, set aside a half-hour and try one of the relaxation techniques given on pages 211–15, followed by one of the suggested visualizations. If you don't find a combination that appeals to you right away, experiment. Use this Pain Emergency Kit as a reference section to which you can return whenever you need to pull another trick out of the hat. Custom-design the information to suit your particular needs: make up your own kit. Embellish this one. Fiddle around with small details.

■ ■ ■

When you are in a pain emergency, you're actually dealing with two separate sets of feelings. One is a high level of physical pain. The other is the sense of panic that inevitably accompanies most emergencies. By addressing the panic first and the pain second, you have the best chance of reducing your pain to a manageable level. This is why the Pain Emergency Kit begins with techniques of relaxation.

Sometimes simply by relaxing your body and concentrating on aspects of your physical self that are *not* feeling pain, you will see your pain diminish within a few minutes. With more severe pain, by first putting yourself into a state of relative calm and diffusing the panic, you can enhance your receptivity, so that the visualizations you use will have a more profound effect.

I like to think of meditation and relaxation techniques as preparing our minds to receive the colorful, imaginative array of visual stimulation that comes with visualization, just as a painter traditionally prepares a canvas for color by first coating it with a layer of white that is called the "ground." For many painters the process of laying the ground is a deeply creative, absorbing act. Just as music needs silence to emerge from and move against, the paint and images need the lead-white "silence" of the ground. Meditation prepares the "ground" of your mind to receive the healing energy of visualizations and other autosuggestive techniques.*

Preparing the Ground: Three Simple Techniques

Most forms of relaxation and meditation use the process of breathing as their focus. Breath is the life force itself; it is the constant interchange between our bodies and the world outside us. It is also a bodily function that continues even when we are unconscious of it, but one which, when consciousness is brought to bear upon it, we can control and often alter in ways that are beneficial to our health. By focusing our awareness on our respiration we can slow it, expand it, deepen it, and even direct the flow of oxygen to certain parts of our bodies. This sort of control is still rudimentary in the West, but in many Eastern cultures the science of breathing has been refined and codified with extraordinary precision and is an accepted, integral part of both religious and medical practice.

Centering   (*Approximate duration: 5–20 minutes*)
This exercise is best done in a quiet, comfortable place and in a seated position. You can sit on the floor, in a chair, or in bed, just so long as you feel comfortable and your back is as straight as possible. Close your eyes and bring your awareness to your breath. You may want to begin by concentrating on the process of inhalation. Inhale slowly and deeply,

---

* The techniques that follow have been culled from many sources. Some are my own, and some have been loosely adapted from other books. Still others were shared with me by health practitioners and the people I interviewed in preparing *The Path to Pain Control*.

preferably with your mouth closed so that you can feel the air passing into your nostrils and down through your pharynx, into your trachea, and finally into your lungs and the tiny pathways of the bronchioles and alveoli. As you exhale, feel your diaphragm rise to help the lungs expel your breath back up through your respiratory tract and out through your nostrils. Some people find it helpful to repeat a simple word or phrase to reinforce their awareness of their breath and keep their mind from wandering. Eastern religions use mantras, special sacred syllables, for this purpose. You can create your own mantra by mentally repeating the same word on each exhalation (a single syllable is easiest — you might try "om" or "peace" or "health"). If extraneous thoughts or images enter your mind, don't judge them. Simply bring your awareness back to the process of your breath, letting your special syllable reinforce your focus.

Head-to-Toe Relaxation *(Approximate duration: 5–10 minutes)*

This exercise is done lying on your back, if possible, on a comfortable surface such as a rug or a mattress. No part of your body should be under particular pressure or stress. With your arms at your side, close your eyes and lie still. Feel your breath moving in and out. Try to focus your awareness on your breath, letting all other thoughts and feelings fall away into peace and silence. Gradually allow your breathing to become deeper, with longer, slower inhalations and even longer exhalations. When you feel comfortable and relaxed, you are ready to embark on a full-length tour of your body, beginning with your feet.

Point your toes and hold. Then relax your feet. Flex your right foot up toward your knee; hold — then let it go. Now do the same with your left foot. Proceed step by step up each side of your body, first right, then left, tensing each major muscle group (calf, thigh, abdominal muscles, buttocks, etc.) and then relaxing it. Make a fist with each hand, then splay your fingers out; hold — and relax. Hunch your shoulders up against your neck; hold — and let them drop back into place. You can even do this with your face. Scrunch your face up tight so that your eyes feel as if they are about to meet your chin; hold — then let your face go slack. Stick your tongue out straight; hold — then let it go and wriggle it around. Shut your eyes tight; hold — then let them open wide and easy. When you've "done the rounds" of your whole body, complete this relaxation exercise by gently shaking yourself loose, letting your head roll, rocking your torso from side to side, and making circles with your feet. (NOTE: If you like, this exercise can be done to music.)

Creating an Energy Flow   (*Approximate duration: 5–10 minutes*)

This exercise can be done either sitting or lying down. With your eyes closed, focus your awareness on your breath as you have done in the two preceding exercises. When you feel ready, continuing to breathe deeply and slowly, shift your awareness to your primary hand (the hand you write with). Without looking at it (your eyes remain closed), simply focus your attention on that hand, as if the rest of your body had dropped away and all your energy had suddenly converged in that hand. Feel its warmth. You may feel its warmth increase, as if there were a sort of glow inside it. With your palm facing down, your hand rests gently, cupping the air inside it.

Now imagine the dial of a clock on the inside of your palm. Very slowly, beginning at 12 o'clock, move your attention to 2 o'clock, inhaling and exhaling slowly and deeply. Keep your focus on that dial, never stopping but continuing to move from one hour to the next as your hand grows warmer and its energy intensifies. You pass 6 o'clock and keep going, gradually moving through 8 o'clock, 9 o'clock and finally to 10. Take the last steps slowly, and when you've come full circle to 12 o'clock, feel the energy that has collected in your hand.

Now take that hand and place it on your chest, letting its warmth penetrate your body. The energy has left your hand and entered a warm spot in the center of your chest. Let it gather there. Now move it, simply by your thoughts, to your left knee. Leave it there and let it penetrate your knee. Move it again, this time to the nape of your neck. Feel the warmth and energy entering that area of your body, removing any tension. Now place your hand behind your neck and recapture the energy, cupping it as before. When your hand is warm, place it on the top of your head and let the energy pour down through your scalp into your whole body. Relax into a few minutes of deep breathing before opening your eyes.

Relaxation Imagery

Once you have begun to relax, you can extend your feeling of peace by adding any one of the following relaxation images. With your eyes still closed, and continuing to inhale deeply and exhale even more deeply, you might want to imagine:

- that you are lying on a billowy cloud, moving gently through space. Feel the texture of the cloud as it buoys you up, and its slow rocking motion. If colors come into your mind, let yourself be surrounded by them. Be held aloft and carried, or simply rest weightless, as you choose. Let yourself be lulled, as if you were in a hammock. Continue to breathe deeply, as your breath becomes one with the breath of the cloud.

- that you are floating on your back in water, staring up at the immense, harmonious blue of a cloudless sky. You may be in a lake, or on the ocean, or lying on a lily pad in a pond. You choose the place. Imagine how it feels to be held and gently moved by the natural flow of water. Let your breath be one with the motion of the water, and fill your eyes with the blue of the sky. See nothing else. If sounds come to you, let them flood your ears. Continue to breathe deeply as you float suspended.

- that you are lying on your stomach in the warm hollow of a sand dune, at peace with yourself and with the elements. Let the sand's heat penetrate your body while the gentle lapping of the nearby waves rocks you into a sleeplike state. Dune grasses fringe you in, swishing softly in the ocean breeze. Each deep breath you take draws in heat; each exhalation brings you closer to the sand's stored energy.

- that you are lying in the cool, high grasses of a fresh green meadow, with a lilting spring breeze rushing over you. In your own hollowed-out hiding place the grass bends down and brushes you, caressing you with long blades that are almost like cool water. Feel the motion of the meadow as it ripples with the wind, a rhythm that is one with the long, peaceful motion of your own relaxed breath. Let yourself be calmed by the sparkling sound of the nearby brook, running full with the first rains of spring.

Techniques That Focus on Your Pain

When you have prepared your "ground" by focusing on your breathing — and perhaps after extending your relaxation through one of the preceding imagery techniques — you may want to focus on the specific area of your body that is most in pain. All of the following are best done while you are still in a relaxed, receptive state, with your eyes closed.

■ Continue to concentrate on the rhythm and pathways of your breath. But this time, as you inhale deeply and exhale even more slowly, imagine that instead of taking air in with your mouth and lungs, you are breathing directly through the area of your body that is hurting. Imagine that this part of you has immediate access to the air outside. Any painful joint, muscle, or internal organ can breathe in and out as if it were a lung. Breathe slowly, maintaining the same pattern of deep breathing that you established in the preceding exercises.

■ Imagine that you are breathing through the soles of your feet, drawing the air up through your legs and into the area of your body that is in pain. Hold your breath there for as long as you can, letting the air circulate freely through the pain, oxygenating the inflamed or injured area. When you exhale, imagine that you are releasing all the pain and tension from that area, along with carbon dioxide. Let each exhalation empty you of pain while each new inhalation brings fresh oxygen to the painful part. You can extend this technique by imagining that the air outside is a healing substance in which you are afloat. Give the outside air any color you want and let that color flood you as you breathe it in. With each inhalation, your body acquires more and more of this healing substance, which it retains, becoming a repository of energy and color. You exhale only the pain.

■ (Especially useful for joint and muscle pain) Lying on your back in bed or on a sofa, imagine that with each inhalation your body slightly rises, and that with each exhalation it sinks gently back. Now visualize your joints, particularly your hips in their sockets, your shoulders in their sockets, your knees, ankles, elbows, and wrists. If your pain is localized, focus your awareness on the area that is causing you most pain. As you inhale, see the joints gently lift in their sockets, floating free of the ligaments and tendons that hold them in place. Hold your breath for as long as you can, giving yourself time to see the suspension you have created in your joints. As you exhale, let the bones settle back into their normal position. Maintain a balanced rhythm of deep inhalations and exhalations for as long as you feel comfortable.

■ Continuing to breathe deeply, imagine that you are sitting outside in a peaceful, comfortable place. I like to think of the pliant, moss-covered earth beneath a willow tree. Now imagine a vertical flow of energy moving down through your whole body into the center of the earth. Concentrate on this flow, letting its motion be the motion of your own deep breathing. As you inhale, draw this life flow up from the center of the earth into your body; as you exhale, send it back through your body down into the earth.

When the flow is established, let it move especially through the part of your body that is most in pain, streaming through that particular area on both inhalation and exhalation. Now imagine that in addition to this flow back and forth between you and the center of the earth there is another flow, one that moves upward from your body to a point infinitely distant in the sky. As you focus your attention on this upward flow, let your breath draw in the energy that emanates from that far-off point. Exhale it back upward with the same rhythm you established while exhaling downward to the center of the earth. When the flow is established, let it move especially through the part of your body that is most in pain, streaming through that particular area on both inhalation and exhalation. Now try to feel both forces simultaneously, so that you are connected to a double flow of healing energy as you continue to breathe slowly and deeply.

Relaxation Imagery Derived from Your Own Pain

The following examples of visualization rely on imagery that in one way or another "takes off" from people's own pain. These tailor-made visualization techniques are often extremely effective. The more you know about the actual physiological processes involved in your own condition, the more detailed you can make your own pain-derived visualizations.

I discovered the potential of pain-derived imagery by chance one night when severe pain was keeping me awake. The painkiller I had taken had had no effect. It was about three o'clock in the morning, and I was lying in the dark, becoming more and more desperate. Suddenly, out of nowhere, came the image of a pitch-black country road at night, going off into the distance. The only light was the white line down the middle of the road. The image presented itself to me complete. I simply followed. I was drawn into a sort of game, in which the object was for me to walk down that center line with the utmost of grace, one foot in front of the other, as if it were a tightrope and I an acrobat. I became thoroughly absorbed in my "craft." There was a sense that if I lost my footing and my foot touched the asphalt on either side of the line, not only would I fall but — somehow even more important in that predawn setting — I would spoil the game. I kept walking, slowly at first, then faster and faster, like a dancer in a trance, exhilarated by the cool evening air and delighted to be speeding into the darkness of a country night. Through this visualization I recaptured my lost sense of speed and grace and — yes, fell asleep! I have returned to it many times at similar moments and found it extremely helpful, reassuring, and relaxing.

Rosalie, whose back sometimes feels as if it is afire (she described her muscles as feeling "raw and flayed"), told me that when her pain is severe she meditates for about ten minutes and then imagines that she is floating on her back in a cool outdoor swimming pool. She is able to maintain this visualization for several minutes at a time. When she feels her attention begin to return to her pain, she simply moves her legs (in her mind) as one must every so often to keep afloat. She has used this visualization to help induce sleep and even to relax at work.

One man I interviewed, who asked to be identified as "Crazy Bob," has severe neck, shoulder, and back pain from an accident at work in which he was struck from behind by a crane. When his pain is at its worst, he feels as if he is locked up in a cage full of tigers. The pain is ferocious, and there is no escape. Thanks to a visualization he uses whenever the pain gets so bad that he can see the tigers, Bob has created his own ingenious escape: "I become an eagle. The image begins with my just seeing the eagle, filling in every detail of his plumage and giving him incredibly beautiful colors. Then at some point I just become him. All of a sudden I'm flying, with this huge wingspan. I see everything down below me — forests, lakes, mountaintops, rivers. It's all so beautiful! And I keep on going, taking it all in. I'm free of the cage of tigers!" Flying and spreading his immense, brightly colored eagle wings, Bob regains the power and vitality his injuries have stripped from him.

A weaver named Anna, cited in Isabel Hanson's *Outwitting Arthritis*, uses her highly developed visual sense to clean her system out when her rheumatoid arthritis acts up. "When there's pain in an arm or leg or other specific place, I often take a trip through my bloodstream, bringing oxygen to that place that needs it and taking away the poisons. Sometimes I just jump in and swim headfirst in the bloodstream with bundles of oxygen in a net behind me, a net with pearls fastened to it. Other times I go on a raft ride. The raft is a red corpuscle, and I sit atop it with my legs crossed and bundles of oxygen within easy reach. First I float up through the heart and lungs to pick up the oxygen, then back down again through the heart to my elbow or knee or wherever. When I get there I toss out a bundle of oxygen and gather in the carbon dioxide, which I get rid of when I ride back up to the lungs."

The Alchemy of Pain: Visualizations That Turn Pain into Non-Pain

As we've seen earlier in *The Path to Pain Control*, particularly in Chapters 2 and 7, the mind has extraordinary powers to transform the life of the body. The images that follow are most effective for getting through short-term medical and dental procedures or for use en route to another visualization. By experimenting with each of them, you may find one that works for you, or you may discover one of your own that isn't listed here.

If your pain follows specific pathways that you can visualize, the next time you're in pain try telling yourself that instead of pain you're feeling:

- filaments of icy water following those paths
- minute trickles of fine sand (as in an hourglass)
- the soft tickle of a feather

If your pain affects a whole area of your body with less clearly defined paths, the next time you're in pain try turning that area into:

- rushing water
- a block of ice
- a honeycomb of light

Another technique is to let go of the rest of your body and see in your mind's eye only the specific pathways or body areas that hurt, as if they were suspended in midair. Let them take on the first color that comes into your imagination. Clearly visualize the patterns traced by your pain in that exact color. Hold that image before your eye. Now switch it to another color — from a warm color to a cool one, or vice versa. Let blue or green become red, orange, or yellow. Let the hot colors turn into their cool opposites. When your painful pathways or body parts have taken on the new color, hold the new image before your eye. When the visualization is clear, switch to a third color. You can keep this one going for as long as you wish, switching from one color to another and even substituting different textures for the anatomical patterns you have traced in your imagination.

Shrinking and Sinking Pain

For pain relief or if you have insomnia because of pain, and counting sheep doesn't work, the following techniques, either separately or combined, may prove especially effective.

In your mind's eye, visualize your pain at its very worst. Let your imagination run wild. Make it as human or inhuman as you like. Deck it out with the strongest adjectives you can, giving it a shape and a height, a color and a texture. Once this image is fixed in your mind, make it ten times the size you originally gave it. Make it gigantic. When this tower-ing, monstrous vision of your very worst pain is as vivid to you as a picture postcard, place it all the way to the left along your mental line of vision. Now move your glance to center field. Leaving the giant where it is, set up a middle-sized version of the same apparition. It looks identical, but shrunken, deflated, and weaker. Let your mind's eye travel back and forth now between the two images of pain, con-scious as you do so that you have shrunk the leftmost monster to the size of the middle one. Your next move is to the right, where a tiny mini-monster, identical to the other two in every respect but size, appears on your imaginary horizon. This third visualization is so small that you almost have to squint to make out its features, even though you know that it is still your pain. By now you have shrunk it to a mere shadow of its former self. (NOTE: For insomnia due to pain, proceed as above, but shrink your pain more grad-ually. Always start with the large economy-size pain on your left and shrink it down by stages as you move to the right.)

Some people find that if they can gather all their pain into one compact, intense red ball, they can temporarily get rid of it by giving it a massive dose of gravity and watching it sink right through the earth, down to the very core, where it either disappears or is buried "forever."

Forms of Distraction

Images With Special Meaning

Several people I interviewed told me that they used com-plicated geometrical designs or imagined every detail of the face of someone they loved in order to distract themselves from feeling pain. One woman whose chronic pain began in early childhood has been using the image of a fondly re-membered oil painting for more than forty years! This painting, a still life of flowers that she describes as "unbelievably corny," hung in the hallway of her parents' home. As a child when she was in pain she used to think of it and be able to fall asleep despite the pain. Now in her sixties, she still finds this image more effective than any other in helping her through her worst bouts of pain.

Fantasy Escapes

A few people possessed of agile imagination are able to distract themselves from pain for hours by imagining themselves in a fantasy situation far removed from where they actually are. I interviewed one woman who said she spends hours in extended daydreams based on the romantic novels she likes to read. She makes herself the heroine and runs the whole plot through her mind, like a movie. She swears by this method of coping with her rheumatoid arthritis.

My own version of a fantasy escape is to return in my mind to places I have loved. I imagine a house I lived in and the exact steps I would have to take to get from my front door to somewhere else. Concentrating on these minute details of memory is often sufficient distraction, when the pain is not too bad, to help me fall asleep. I particularly love returning to Venice, where I lived for a year before I got sick, with its labyrinth of streets and canals.

Laughter

Reading humorous stories or watching funny movies can be one of the all-time best escapes from pain. But laughter goes beyond mere distraction. In *Anatomy of an Illness* Norman Cousins describes his conscious use of laughter, along with intravenous vitamin C, to reverse the effects of a serious collagen disease. According to Cousins, "Illness is not a laughing matter. Perhaps it ought to be. Laughter is a form of internal jogging. It moves your internal organs around. It enhances respiration. It is an igniter of great expectations." I put this notion to the test on a recent plane trip. I was in intense pain. Unable to concentrate on the book I had brought along, I succumbed to the offer of a set of plastic headphones and tuned in to what turned out to be an hour's worth of stand-up comedy on tape. I laughed myself silly, and when the tape was done my pain was almost gone.

The Power of the Word

I have already mentioned the Eastern tradition of mantras, or words used in ritual practices such as meditation. Many people, quite independently of these traditions, have found a special word or phrase that calms them when they are in pain. You may have already discovered one that works for you. If not, perhaps the following examples will give you some ideas.

Immanuel Kant, the German philosopher who spent his life pondering the great questions of existence, was plagued by gout in his old age. In a letter to a friend he wrote, "One night, impatient at being kept awake by pain, I availed myself of the stoical means of concentration upon some indifferent object of thought, such for instance as the name of 'Cicero' with its multifarious associations; in this way I found it possible to divert my attention, so that the pain was soon dulled ... Whenever the attacks recur and disturb my sleep, I find this remedy most useful."

A French professor told me that she uses a treasured line from the nineteenth-century poet Baudelaire to take the edge off severe pain. The sounds themselves are soothing, and for her they work as a kind of charm or incantation: "*Soi sage, ô ma douleur, et tiens-toi plus tranquille*" (Be good, oh my pain, and calm thyself).

Some of the people I interviewed used simple statements that served as a direct message to their pain:

- "You're fading, fading, fading. You are disappearing out of sight."
- "Every day, in every way, I'm feeling better."

Pain Countdown

This final exercise is based on the Plain Ordinary Pain Scale presented on page 34, where 1 is the least amount of pain you've ever felt and 10 is the worst pain you can imagine. Wherever you are when you begin this countdown visualization, be sure you are relaxed and that you are in a place where you can remain with your eyes closed for several minutes. Begin by determining your pain level on the Plain Ordinary Pain Scale. Now visualize the scale stretched out before you as if it were the whole horizon. Place an imaginary line at the point that indicates your present level of pain. Let's say it's 8. *Very* slowly, letting your eyes move from right to left, move your pain from 8 to 7. Hold it there. Inhale and exhale slowly and deeply. Now begin to subdivide. Very slowly, once again, letting your eyes move from right to left, move your pain from 7 to 6½. Hold it there. Inhale and exhale slowly and deeply. Continue another half-step, moving your pain from 6½ to 6. At this point you may have reduced your pain to the point where you wish to try a different visualization. If not, keep going, but move as slowly as you can, reducing your pain by half-counts and then by quarter-counts for as long as you can or until you fall asleep. (This technique is very effective for insomnia.) The opposite of this is the classic wisdom of the writer Henry de Montherlant: "You can dull the edge of any pain by imagining how much worse it could be."

Notes
Techniques that have worked best for me are:

Afterword

The path to pain control is not a journey with a destination or an end; having read this far, you have not "arrived." But you are well on your way. You've worked hard through the pages of this book, and it is my hope that you will come away from it with a clear vision of your own path to pain control. You know now that this path is a process, a way of living with pain and learning from it over time. Your relationship to pain is constantly changing, but with the tools for awareness you now possess, you are well equipped to continue on your own.

 If you return to this book from time to time, you may find that certain aspects of it no longer seem important, while others have taken on a new significance. This will be because you have not stood still. Life moves, you move, pain moves. Issues that are issues for you now will have been resolved. And as you continue on your path you will meet the challenges that arise with the sure knowledge that pain doesn't have to be something you just react to: it can be a catalyst that leads to pain reduction and control, a catalyst for change.

Coping Resource Guide
Suggested Reading List
Bibliography
Index

Coping Resource Guide*

Alternative Therapies for Pain

Acupuncture

Acupuncture is an ancient Chinese treatment with a five-thousand-year history of practice and erudite development throughout the East. As Dr. David Bresler, director of the U.C.L.A. Pain Control Unit, writes, "although some American physicians still consider acupuncture to be 'experimental,' more people have probably been treated with it than all other systems of medicine combined."

Following body pathways known as "meridians," acupuncture uses hair-thin stainless steel needles to activate the currents of energy that Chinese medicine believes to be the active principle in both health and disease. Much of the success of acupuncture treatment depends on the acupuncturist's skill in assessing which of hundreds of specific points on the meridians need to be used, as well as the proper placement and insertion of the needles. Many acupuncturists

* Wherever possible national addresses have been given. Most groups listed will supply names and addresses of chapters or similar organizations near where you live.

believe that the manipulation of the needles by twirling them by hand or by applying electricity or heat can enhance the effect of the treatment.

For most chronic pain problems, a series of treatments is needed to determine whether acupuncture will work at all. Thus, you have to be willing to give it a try and not expect instantaneous results. However, if there is no effect whatsoever after about ten sessions, a responsible practitioner should recommend that you discontinue the treatment.

Both here and in the East there is a range of approaches to acupuncture. In this country, generally speaking, the major differences hinge on how traditional or how Westernized the practice is. Many Western physicians believe that the Chinese meridian charts have no basis in established physiology and do not follow them. Traditional practitioners, many of them born or trained in China, sometimes accuse American health professionals who practice acupuncture of latching onto an ancient, intricate science without fully understanding it, of distorting it, of lacking the proper finesse in inserting the needles, and so forth.

With these differences and disputes in mind, I've listed information sources for both Westernized and traditional acupuncture. If you are considering acupuncture you need to follow your own bent in choosing a practitioner whose views most match your own. There are quacks galore in this field, on both sides of the fence. In acupuncture's favor, however, is the fact that it is unlikely to have any harmful effects. If it works for you, you're in luck; and if not, you shouldn't be any worse off than you were before. Two points to keep in mind: (1) Be sure you understand the full cost of any treatment you undertake. Most insurance companies will not reimburse for acupuncture unless it is given by a licensed M.D. (2) Acupuncture is not generally viewed as a method of cure. It can, however, provide extended periods of relief from pain.

Further information on acupuncture, and names of practitioners in your area, can be obtained from:

American Association of Acupuncture and Oriental Medicine
4400 East-West Highway
Suite 1030
Bethesda, Maryland 20814

Biofeedback

Biofeedback is a child of the computer age. The term refers to the feedback, or flow of information, from the body onto the TV-like screen of various computer terminals and other devices that show graphically what is going on inside the body. Many functions of which we are normally unaware, such as temperature, pulse, blood pressure, and muscle tension, can be projected onto these screens through the use of electrodes placed on the skin. The theory behind all the wires and space-age lights and blips is that by getting a continuous, instantaneous flow of information, you can learn to control certain body functions that were previously considered inaccessible to voluntary change. Biofeedback has been used most effectively to control migraine, high blood pressure, and muscle tension associated with neck and lower back pain.

Biofeedback works hand in hand with techniques of relaxation and meditation such as those described in the Pain Emergency Kit. The main difference is that with biofeedback you actually see whether and how much you are relaxing and whether you are relaxing the area(s) in your body that need it most. Once the basic concepts have been mastered through the use of the machines, the assumption is that patients retain the relaxation skills and can continue on their own without equipment.

Most clinics and hospitals have biofeedback training programs. A number of private practitioners also give biofeedback training, including psychologists, psychotherapists, psychiatrists, and physical therapists, who sometimes offer it in conjunction with other forms of therapy. Again, as with acupuncture, be sure to check on cost before you begin a course of treatment. If biofeedback is not "rendered" by an M.D., you may have trouble with insurance. If you are unable to find a biofeedback training program in your area (check the Yellow Pages), you can get a local referral by writing to:

Biofeedback Society of America
4301 Owens Street
Wheatridge, Colorado 80033
(303) 422–8436

Hypnosis and Self-Hypnosis

Hypnosis for the treatment of pain has little to do with the stage tricks many people still associate with it. Hypnosis is a state of relaxation (not unlike meditation) in which you are particularly receptive and attentive to suggestion. The suggestion can be in the form of verbal messages ("I feel less pain with each breath I take") or visual images ("My back is relaxed and supple, I'm running on the edge of the beach"), and it can be "planted" by a trained hypnotist or by you yourself once you have learned how. Like biofeedback training, hypnosis for pain control often requires several sessions. Ideally, self-hypnosis should be the goal of these sessions, so that you will be able to integrate hypnosis into your daily life. The basic techniques can be learned fairly quickly, but they do require constant practice if they are to remain effective. Many people find that hypnosis learned for one purpose, such as pain control, has many other applications in their lives. Hypnosis can be used to enhance concentration, combat nervousness, reduce stage fright, defuse anger, and so forth.

Hypnotists are listed in the Yellow Pages of most major

cities. The usual caveats about cost and quacks apply. You might want to check with a local medical center for a hypnotist with extensive experience in treating chronic pain. For reliable referrals contact:

American Society for Clinical
  Hypnosis
2400 East Devon Avenue
Des Plaines, Illinois 60018
(312) 297-3317

Society for Clinical and
  Experimental Hypnosis
129A King's Park Drive
Liverpool, New York 13088
(315) 652-7299
(send a stamped, self-addressed envelope)

Pain Clinics

Pain clinics are essentially a phenomenon of the past ten years, although a handful go back further than that. They are multidisciplinary centers that focus exclusively on the treatment of pain, regardless of its medical origin. This means that under one roof you may find neurosurgeons, psychologists, orthopedists, rheumatologists, physical therapists, psychiatrists, dentists, social workers, and nurses, any of whom can be called in to collaborate in diagnosing and treating a specific patient.

At this point there are over four hundred pain clinics in the United States, with more opening every year. Their main success seems to be defined by both health professionals and clinic "graduates" in terms of *education;* that is, patients who complete these programs (usually three to six weeks on an inpatient basis) learn that there are many ways to approach chronic pain and that it is possible to live a full life even with some degree of pain. Individual and group psychotherapy are important components of many of these programs. Another major orientation — accounting for up to 65 percent of treatment, according to some estimates — is drug detoxification; a large percentage of pain clinic patients are dependent on painkillers and tranquilizers. To date, no significant follow-up studies have been produced by any of the leading pain clinics.

Pain clinics are probably best able to help those who feel that their pain has become hopelessly entangled with other difficult aspects of their lives. Being on a ward with other patients in the same situation and exploring some of the key issues that affect everyone with pain often helps to clarify where pain leaves off and other problems begin, opening the way for therapeutic change — for example, the resolution of marital tensions, vocational frustration, and so forth.

A number of major medical centers have pain clinics. Most, but not all, are residential, inpatient programs. Outpatient programs do exist but are more common in the private sector. Although the cost of all pain clinics is extremely high, many insurance policies, as well as workmen's compensation, will pay some of the bills. If you are considering becoming a pain clinic patient, be sure to get full financial information from both the clinic and your insurance company before signing yourself in. Some insurance carriers will pay room and board but not all medical costs; some draw the line at psychotherapy and vocational counseling.

Reliable referrals can be obtained from:

American Pain Society
New York University Medical Center
550 First Avenue
New York, New York 10016
(212) 340–6623

Self-Help
Self-help groups for people with chronic pain can provide an invaluable source of support. Members get together once or twice a month to share ideas, to hear speakers on topics of interest, and often to hold social gatherings that include family and friends. Very few of these groups exist as of this

writing, but you might want to take the lead and form one in your own community or neighborhood. Guidelines on doing this are available from:

Pain Copers, Inc.
125 Nashua Street
Boston, Massachusetts 02114
(send a stamped, self-addressed envelope)

General Community Services

If you are in need of a particular service and are not sure of where to go or how to proceed, contact the mayor's office, the office of your representative in Congress, or religious and civic groups in your immediate community. Even if they can't answer all your questions, they should be able to point you in the right direction.

Adult Education

Many school systems offer courses in a broad range of skills and subjects. Check with your local school board or write to:

Adult Education Association
1225 19th Street, N.W.
Washington, D.C. 20036

Legal Services

Most telephone directories will list an office of Legal Aid or some other form of legal assistance. For national information check the organizations listed on pages 240–42 under "Special Interest Groups."

Nursing
Most communities have a local Visiting Nurses Association.

Psychotherapy
The best sources for referral are a local medical center or friends whose opinions and recommendations you are inclined to trust.

Transportation
Many communities have reduced bus and subway fares for the elderly and the disabled. For van services, check with your physician or medical center.

Vocational Counseling and/or Rehabilitation
Vocational counseling is available to those receiving Social Security disability payments or workmen's compensation through the Office of Vocational Rehabilitation (OVR), which is organized by state. Check with your local Social Security Office for precise information. Many health professionals such as social workers and career counselors offer vocational guidance either privately or through existing clinics. Check your Yellow Pages under "Career," "Counseling," and "Vocational."

Health Activist Groups

- American Coalition of Citizens with Disabilities
  1346 Connecticut Avenue, N.W.
  Washington, D.C. 20036
  (202) 785-4256

■ Gray Panthers National Health Service Task Force
3700 Chestnut Street
Philadelphia, Pennsylvania 19004
(215) 382–3300

■ Health Policy Advisory Center (Health/PAC)
217 Murray Street
New York, New York 10007
(212) 267–8890
"A network for health activists to discuss, share, and analyze their concerns and strategies with others across the country engaged in similar endeavors"; publishes the *Health/PAC Bulletin*.

Medical Consumer Groups

■ Center for Medical Consumers and Health Care
Information, Inc.
237 Thompson Street
New York, New York 10012
(212) 674–7105
"An alternate source of health information," offering free medical library open to the public and a phone-in tape service on a wide range of medical subjects, and serving as a clearinghouse for health information.
Publishes bimonthly newsletter, *Health Facts*.

■ Public Citizens Health Research Group
2000 P Street, N.W.
Washington, D.C. 20036
(202) 872–0320
An activist and research group "fighting for the public's health in Washington, and giving consumers more control over decisions which affect their health."
Extensive list of publications available on request, including two of special interest to readers of this book:

Getting Yours: A Consumer's Guide to Obtaining Your Medical Records ($2.50)

Your Money or Your Health, a guide to getting the most out of Medicare: geared to people sixty-five or over ($4.00)

Special Interest Groups

Disabled

■ Disability Rights Center
1346 Connecticut Avenue, N.W.
Washington, D.C. 20036
(202) 223-3304

■ Center for Independent Living
2539 Telegraph Avenue
Berkeley, California 94704
(415) 841-4776
An activist-oriented center staffed primarily by disabled people, providing a range of services including group and peer counseling; advice and assistance relating to education, employment, housing and equipment; legal counsel and general advocacy; and outreach on issues that affect the disabled. Publishes the *Independent,* a quarterly magazine. The Berkeley C.I.L. is the prototype for a number of similar centers throughout the country. They keep a complete regional directory and will give you information on a center near you.

Senior Citizens

■ The Gray Panthers
3635 Chestnut Street
Philadelphia, Pennsylvania 19104
(215) 382-3300

- National Council on Aging
  1848 L Street, N.W., Suite 504
  Washington, D.C. 20036
  (202) 223-6250

- National Senior Citizens Law Center
  1424 16th Street, N.W., Suite 300
  Washington, D.C. 20036
  (202) 232-6570

Veterans

- Paralyzed Veterans of America
  4350 East-West Highway, Suite 900
  Bethesda, Maryland 20014
  (301) 652-2135

- Vietnam Veterans of America
  212 Fifth Avenue
  New York, New York 10003
  (212) 685-3152

- Vietnam Veterans Outreach Centers
  A newly formed network of informal counseling centers
  throughout the U.S. (check with VA).

Women

Many cities and towns across the country list women's
bookstores and women's centers in their phone books;
both are good sources of information on women's health
groups and related activities.

- National Women's Health Network
  224 Seventh Street, S.E.
  Washington, D.C. 20003
  (202) 543-9222

■ Coalition for the Medical Rights of Women
1638B Haight Street
San Francisco, California 94117
(415) 621–8030

Suggested Reading List

All titles are available in paperback. Books marked with an asterisk are those I recommend as particularly encouraging for anybody faced with a chronic medical condition.

Herbert Benson, *The Relaxation Response* (Avon, 1976).
An excellent introduction to the concept of mind-body integration. Presents one of the simplest, most basic forms of meditation.

Richard Nelson Bolles, *What Color Is Your Parachute?* (Ten Speed Press, 1980).
A job hunter's manual with a twist: shows you how to find the job that needs *you*. Excellent reference section.

* Eric J. Cassell, *The Healer's Art* (Penguin, 1979).
A thoughtful look at the doctor-patient relationship by a practicing internist. Especially insightful on the impact of chronic illness.

* Colette, *The Blue Lantern*, translated by Roger Senhouse (Farrar, Straus & Giroux, 1963).
Autobiography and reminiscences by the great French novelist, written when she was in her mid-seventies and bedridden with arthritis. A passionate response to pain and disability.

Gena Corea, *The Hidden Malpractice* (Jove, 1978).
An impressively documented exploration of how American medicine treats women, both as patients and as professionals.

* Norman Cousins, *Anatomy of an Illness* (Bantam, 1981).
  A stimulating, well-argued collection of essays by the editor emeritus of the *Saturday Review*. Illuminates the importance of the author's active participation in bringing about his eventual recovery from a crippling collagen disease.

Joe Graedon, *The People's Pharmacy* (Avon, 1977) and *The People's Pharmacy 2* (Avon, 1980).
  Excellent, fact-packed guides to prescription drugs.

Isabel Hanson, *Outwitting Arthritis* (Creative Arts Book Company, 1980).
  A collection of interviews with people who have arthritis, with an emphasis on individual solutions to the problems of the most common chronic illness.

Ivan Illich, *Medical Nemesis* (Bantam, 1977).
  A provocative attack on the medical system as we know it; brilliantly argued and researched.

Peter Parish, *The Doctors' and Patients' Handbook of Medicines and Drugs* (Alfred A. Knopf, 1980).
  An excellent reference book on prescription and nonprescription drugs; for those who want a detailed understanding of how drugs work.

* Susan Sontag, *Illness as Metaphor* (Vintage, 1980).
  An imaginative essay on how society views illness; Sontag argues that the healthiest way of being ill is that least burdened by complex, often punitive interpretations.

Shunryu Suzuki, *Zen Mind, Beginner's Mind* (Weatherhill, 1980).
  A collection of short essays by the late Zen master. One of the best introductions to the Zen Buddhist way of looking at life.

John White and Richard Fadiman, eds., *Relax* (Dell, 1976).
  An excellent anthology of relaxation and meditation techniques; if you have this book you can dispense with about twenty others.

Especially for Health Professionals:

David Brandon, *Zen in the Art of Helping* (Delta, 1976).
  An innovative, reflective, challenging approach to the helping professions by a British social worker.

Anselm Strauss and Barney Glaser, *Chronic Illness and the Quality of Life* (C. V. Mosby, 1976).
A perceptive analysis of the American health care system in relation to the problems of chronic illness.

Bibliography

(Does not include titles that appear on the
Suggested Reading List)

Beaver, William T., "Mild Analgesics: A Review of Their Clinical Pharmacology." *American Journal of the Medical Sciences,* 250 (5); 577–599, 1965.

Beecher, Henry K., "Pain in Men Wounded in Battle." *Annals of Surgery,* 123:96, 1946.

Benson, Herbert, *The Mind/Body Effect.* New York: Simon and Schuster, 1979.

Benson, H., and D. P. McCallie, Jr., "Angina Pectoris and the Placebo Effect." *New England Journal of Medicine,* 300:1424–1429, 1979.

Bonica, John J., *The Management of Pain.* Philadelphia: Lea and Febiger, 1953.

Brena, Steven F., ed., *Chronic Pain: America's Hidden Epidemic.* New York: Atheneum, 1978.

———, *Pain and Religion: A Psychophysiological Study.* Springfield, Illinois: Charles C Thomas, 1972.

———, *Yoga and Medicine.* New York: Julian Press, 1972.

Bresler, David E., *Free Yourself from Pain.* New York: Simon and Schuster, 1979.

Buss, A. H., and N. W. Portnoy, "Pain Tolerance and Group Identification." *Journal of Personality and Social Psychology,* 6 (1): 106–108, 1967.

Cassell, Eric J., "Changing Ideas of Causality in Medicine."
Social Research, 46 (4):728–743, 1979.

Chapman, C. Richard, and Ronald Melzack, "Psychological Aspects of Pain." *Postgraduate Medicine*, 53 (6): 69–75, 1973.

Clark, J. W., and D. Bindra, "Individual Differences in Pain Threshold." *Canadian Journal of Psychology*, 10:69–76, 1956.

Clark, W. Crawford, "Pain Sensitivity and the Report of Pain." In M. Weisenberg and B. Tursky, eds., *Pain: New Perspectives in Therapy and Research*. New York: Plenum Press, 1976.

———, and Susanne Bennett, "Pain Responses in Nepalese Porters." *Science*, 209:410–411, 1980.

Cooperstock, Ruth, "A Review of Women's Psychotropic Drug Use." *Canadian Journal of Psychiatry*, 24:29–34, 1979.

Critchley, M., "Congenital Indifference to Pain." *Annals of Internal Medicine*, 45:737, 1956.

Degenaar, J. J., "Some Philosophical Considerations on Pain." *Pain*, 7:281–304, 1979.

Dick-Read, Grantly, *Childbirth Without Fear*. New York: Dell, 1962 (original, 1944).

Dougherty, Ronald J., "Transcutaneous Electrical Nerve Stimulation: An Alternative to Drugs in the Treatment of Chronic Pain." Paper delivered at the meeting of the American Pain Society, New York, September 1980.

Ebert, Robert H., "Medical Education in the United States." In John Knowles, ed., *Doing Better and Feeling Worse*. New York: W. W. Norton, 1977.

Eisenberg, Leon, "The Search for Care." In John Knowles, ed., *Doing Better and Feeling Worse*. New York: W. W. Norton, 1977.

Fabrega, H. J., et al., "Culture, Language, and the Shaping of Illness: An Illustration Based on Pain." *Journal of Psychosomatic Research*, 20 (4):323–337, 1976.

Fairley, Peter, *The Conquest of Pain*. New York: Scribner's, 1980.

Flach, Frederic F., *Choices*. New York: Bantam, 1979.

Folkard, S., et al., "Diurnal Variation and Individual Differences in the Perception of Intractable Pain." *Journal of Psychosomatic Research*, 20:289–301, 1976.

Fox, Renee C., "The Medicalization and Demedicalization of American Society." In John Knowles, ed., *Doing Better and Feeling Worse*. New York: W. W. Norton, 1977.

Freedman, Lawrence Z., and Verna M. Ferguson, "The Question of 'Painless' Childbirth in Primitive Cultures." *American Journal of Orthopsychiatry*, 20 (2):363–372, 1950.

Freese, Arthur S., *Pain*. New York: Penguin, 1975.

Fries, James F., *Arthritis: A Comprehensive Guide*. Reading, Massachusetts: Addison-Wesley, 1979.

Fülöp-Miller, René, *Triumph over Pain*. New York: Literary Guild, 1938.

Gelb, Harold, *Killing Pain Without Prescription*. New York: Harper and Row, 1980.

Gonda, T. A., "The Relation Between Complaints of Persistent Pain and Family Size." *Journal of Neurology, Neurosurgery, and Psychology*, 25:277–281, 1962.

Goolkasian, Paula, "Cyclic Changes in Pain Perception." *Perception and Psychophysics*, 27 (6):499–504, 1980.

Graham, David T., "Health, Disease, and the Mind-Body Problem: Linguistic Parallels." *Psychosomatic Medicine*, 29:52–71, 1967.

Hannington-Kiff, John G., *Pain Relief*. London: Heinemann, 1974.

Harkins, W. W., "Age and Sex Differences in Pain Perception." In D. J. Anderson and B. Mathews, eds., *Pain in Trigeminal Region*. New York: Elsevier North-Holland, 1977.

Hendler, Nelson H., and Judith A. Fenton, *Coping with Chronic Pain*. New York: Clarkson Potter, 1979.

Hilgard, Ernest R., and Josephine R. Hilgard, *Hypnosis in the Relief of Pain*. Los Altos, California: W. Kaufmann, 1975.

Hill, Harris, et al., "Studies on Anxiety Associated with the Anticipation of Pain." *Archives of Neurology and Psychiatry*, 67:612–619, 1952.

Houde, Raymond W., "Medical Treatment of Oncological Pain." In J. Bonica, P. Procacci, and C. A. Pagni, eds., *Recent Advances in Pain: Pathophysiology and Clinical Aspects*. Springfield, Illinois: Charles C Thomas, 1974.

———, "Principles of Clinical Management." In H. W. Kosterlitz and L. Y. Terenius, eds., *Pain and Society*. Weinheim: Verlag Chemie, 1980.

Jong, R. H., "Central Pain Mechanisms." *Journal of the American Medical Association*, 239 (26):2784, 1978.

Knowles, John H., ed., *Doing Better and Feeling Worse: Health in the United States*. New York: W. W. Norton, 1977.

Kruger, Helen, *Other Healers, Other Cures.* New York: Bobbs-Merrill, 1974.

Lack, Dorothea Z., "Pain and the Female Patient." Paper presented at the meeting of the American Pain Society, New York, September 1980.

Lasagna, Louis, "The Clinical Evaluation of Morphine and Its Substitutes as Analgesics." *Pharmacological Review,* 16:47–83, 1964.

Levine, J. D., N. O. Gordon, and H. L. Fields, "The Mechanism of Placebo Analgesia." *Lancet,* September 23, 1978, pp. 654–657.

Melzack, Ronald, *The Puzzle of Pain.* New York: Harper Torchbooks, 1973.

———, and T. H. Scott, "Effects of Early Experience on the Response to Pain." *Journal of Comparative Physiology and Psychology,* 50:155, 1957.

Merskey, H., and D. Boyd, "Emotional Adjustments and Chronic Pain." *Pain,* 5:173–178, 1978.

———, and G. D. Watson, "The Lateralization of Pain." *Pain,* 7:271–280, 1979.

Mines, Samuel, *The Conquest of Pain.* New York: Grosset and Dunlap, 1974.

Neal, Helen, *The Politics of Pain.* New York: McGraw-Hill, 1978.

Parker, Gail Thain, *Mind Cure in New England.* Hanover, New Hampshire: University Press of New England, 1973.

Pawlicki, Robert E., "Demographic and Behavioral Factors Amongst Chronic Pain Patients from a Rural Appalachian Setting." Paper presented at the meeting of the American Pain Society, New York, September 1980.

Pelletier, Kenneth R., *Mind as Healer, Mind as Slayer.* New York: Delta, 1977.

Poznanski, Elva O., "Children's Reactions to Pain: A Psychiatrist's Perspective." *Clinical Pediatrics,* 15(12):114–119, 1976.

Procacci, P., et al., "Studies on the Pain Threshold in Man." In *Advances in Neurology,* vol. 4. New York: Raven Press, 1974.

Reuler, James B., Donald D. Girard, and David A. Nardone, "The Chronic Pain Syndrome: Misconceptions and Management." *Annals of Internal Medicine,* 3 (4):588–596, 1980.

Rogers, Ada G., "Pharmacology of Analgesics." *Journal of Neurosurgical Nursing,* 10(4):180–184, 1978.

Seligman, M. E. P., and G. Beagley, "Learned Helplessness in the Rat." *Journal of Comparative Physiology and Psychology,* 88:534–541, 1975.

Selye, Hans, *The Stress of Life.* New York: McGraw-Hill, 1956.

Shanfield, Stephen B., Elliott M. Heiman, D. Nathan Cope, and John R. Jones, "Pain and the Marital Relationship: Psychiatric Distress." *Pain,* 7:343–351, 1979.

Shipman, W. G., et al., "Correlation of Placebo Response and Personality Characteristics in Myofascial Pain Dysfunction." *Journal of Psychosomatic Research,* 18:475, 1974.

Simonton, O. Carl, and Stephanie Matthews Simonton, *Getting Well Again.* New York: Bantam, 1980.

Steinberg, Milton, *Basic Judaism.* New York: Harcourt Brace Jovanovich, 1947.

Sternbach, Richard A., *Pain: A Psychophysiological Analysis.* New York: Academic Press, 1968.

————, *Pain Patients: Traits and Treatments.* New York: Academic Press, 1974.

Strauss, Anselm, and Barney Glaser, *The Discovery of Grounded Theory.* New York: Aldine, 1967.

Szasz, Thomas, "The Psychology of Persistent Pain." In A. Soulairac, ed., *Pain.* London: Academic Press, 1968.

Thomas, Lewis, "On the Science and Technology of Medicine." In John Knowles, ed., *Doing Better and Feeling Worse.* New York: W. W. Norton, 1977.

Totman, Richard, *The Social Causes of Illness.* New York: Pantheon, 1980.

Tursky, Bernard, "The Development of a Pain Perception Profile: A Psychophysiological Approach." In M. Weisenberg and B. Tursky, eds., *Pain: New Perspectives in Therapy and Research.* New York: Plenum Press, 1976.

Vogel, Albert V., James S. Goodwin, and Jean M. Goodwin, "The Therapeutics of Placebo." *Annals of Family Practice,* July 1980, pp. 105–109.

Von Graffenrild, B., et al., "The Influence of Anxiety and Pain Sensitivity on Experimental Pain in Man." *Pain,* 4 (3):253–263, 1978.

Weisenberg, M., ed., *Pain: Clinical and Experimental Perspectives.* St. Louis, Missouri: C. V. Mosby, 1975.

Wolf, Barbara, *Living with Pain.* New York: Seabury Press, 1977.

Wolff, B. B., and A. A. Horland, "The Effect of Suggestion upon Experimental Pain: A Validation Study." *Journal of Abnormal Psychology*, 72:402–407, 1967.

———, and S. Langley, "Cultural Factors and the Responses to Pain." *American Anthropologist*, 70:494, 1968.

Woodrow, Kenneth M., et al., "Pain Tolerance: Differences According to Age, Sex, and Race." In M. Weisenberg, ed., *Pain: Clinical and Experimental Perspectives*. St. Louis, Missouri: C. V. Mosby, 1975.

Woolf, Virginia, "On Being Ill." In *The Moment and Other Essays*. New York: Harvest Books, 1974 (original, London, 1947).

Zborowski, Mark, "Cultural Components in Responses to Pain." *Journal of Social Issues*, 8:16, 1952.

———, *People in Pain*. San Francisco: Jossey-Bass, 1969.

Index

Medications. *See* Drug(s)
Meditation, 23, 95, 210–11
Melzack, Ronald, *The Puzzle of Pain*, 17–18
Memoirs of John Abernethy, The, 93
Memorial Sloan-Kettering Institute for Cancer Research, Analgesic Studies Section at, 150
Men, effects of social stereotypes on medical treatment of, 74–77
Menstruation, difficult, 5
Migraine headaches, 5, 95, 149, 169–70
Miltown (meprobamate), 149
Mind: and body, interaction of, to create and control pain, 16, 49–50; -body research, 17–19; housecleaning of, 32–33; and placebo effect, 19–21
Model of pain behavior: negative, 6–7; replacing, 12–13
Monoamine oxidase (MAO) inhibitor group of antidepressants, 165
Montherlant, Henry de, 226
Morphine, 18, 155, 161, 163, 164; and endorphins, 21–23
Morrison, Toni, *The Bluest Eye*, 68
Motrin (ibuprofen), 149
Multiple sclerosis, 5, 170
Muscle relaxants, 149
Myasthenia gravis, 5
Myofascial syndrome, 5

Naloxone, 22
Naprosyn (naproxen), 149

National Arthritis Foundation, 85
National Center for Health Statistics, 85
National Press Club, 154
Neal, Helen, 5
Nembutal (pentobarbital), 149
Nepalese, pain tolerance of, 78–79
Nerve blocks, 15
New England Journal of Medicine, 20
New York University, 19
Nitroglycerin, 149
"Noxious stimulus," 16
Nursing services, 238
Nutrition, influence on pain of, 57–60

"Old American" (WASP), attitudes toward pain of, 80, 81
Opiates, 155
Opium, 161
Osler, William, 65, 147
Osteoarthritis, 5
Oxycodone, 149, 163

Pain, chronic: acute vs., 9–11; age and, 89–91; *aikido* response to, 117–19, 120, 121, 123, 125, 129, 176, 200; alchemy of, 114–16, 220–21; alternative therapies for, 231–37; bodily awareness and, 97–98; clinics, 235–36; compounders, 45–46, 47, 200; conditioning about, 5–6; conditions causing, 4–5; consequences of, 11–

Author's Note

If *The Path to Pain Control* has helped you, you can help others with chronic pain by sharing your reactions, as well as your own tried and true techniques for coping, by writing to me. Your comments, criticisms, and contributions will help ensure that future editions of this book accurately reflect both the needs and the wisdom of people with chronic pain. Confidentiality and anonymity will be strictly respected where requested.

All correspondence may be sent to:

> Meg Bogin
> c/o Houghton Mifflin Company
> 2 Park Street
> Boston, Massachusetts 02108